# Here's How to Do Accent Modification: A Manual for Speech-Language Pathologists

# "Here's How"

Thomas Murry, PhD
*Series Editor*

*Here's How to Do Therapy: Hands-On Core Skills in Speech-Language Pathology, Second Edition* by Debra M. Dwight, EdD

*Here's How to Treat Dementia* by Jennifer L. Loehr, MA, CCC-SLP and Megan L. Malone, MA, CCC-SLP

*Here's How to Provide Intervention for Children with Autism Spectrum Disorder: A Balanced Approach* by Catherine B. Zenko, MS, CCC-SLP and Michelle Peters Hite, MS, CCC-SLP

*Here's How to Do Early Intervention for Speech and Language: Empowering Parents* by Karyn Lewis Searcy, MA, CCC-SLP

*Here's How to Do Stuttering Therapy* by Gary J. Rentschler, PhD

*Here's How Children Learn Speech and Language: A Text on Different Learning Strategies* by Margo Kinzer Courter, MA, CCC-SLP

*Here's How to Treat Childhood Apraxia of Speech, Second Edition* by Margaret Fish, MS, CCC-SLP

*Here's How to Teach Voice and Communication Skills to Transgender Women* by Abbie Olszewski, PhD, CCC-SLP, Selah Sullivan, MS, CCC-SLP, and Adriano Cabral, MFA

# Here's How to Do Accent Modification: A Manual for Speech-Language Pathologists

Robert McKinney, MA, CCC-SLP

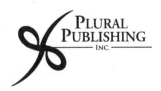

PLURAL
PUBLISHING
INC.

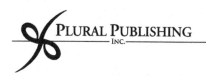

5521 Ruffin Road
San Diego, CA 92123

e-mail: information@pluralpublishing.com
Web site: https://www.pluralpublishing.com

Typeset in 11/15 Stone Informal by Achorn International
Printed in the United States of America by Integrated Books International
24  23  22  21      3  4  5  6

Library of Congress Cataloging-in-Publication Data
Names: McKinney, Robert (Speech-language pathologist), author.
Title: Here's how to do accent modification : a manual for speech-language
   pathologists / Robert McKinney.
Description: San Diego, CA : Plural Publishing, [2019] | Includes
   bibliographical references and index.
Identifiers: LCCN 2018055066| ISBN 9781635500073 (alk. paper) |
   ISBN 1635500079 (alk. paper)
Subjects: | MESH: Language Therapy—methods | Language Development
Classification: LCC RC423 | NLM WL 340.3 | DDC 616.85/5206—dc23
LC record available at https://lccn.loc.gov/2018055066

# Contents

# Introduction

"I've been working as a speech-language pathologist for several years now, but I'm interested in changing it up a little and have been looking into getting involved in accent modification. I know it's part of our scope of practice, but it's a foreign area to me and I have no idea where to begin. I would like to take some trainings and buy some materials for help. Any tips on how or where to start? Any information would be greatly appreciated!"

—Anonymous

Those of us working in the world of accent modification have heard variations on this question throughout our careers. I wrote this book to answer it. *Here's How to Do Accent Modification* is designed primarily for speech-language pathologists (SLPs) looking to bridge the gap between the insights and techniques they have developed in their work with communicative disorders and the skills and knowledge that will help them excel with clients whose communication challenges are related to language differences. It is also aimed at graduate clinicians and supervisors who work on accents, and it provides a fresh perspective to those who come to the field with other backgrounds, such as teachers of English to speakers of other languages, and voice and speech trainers. There is an emphasis on practical tips, techniques, and examples, and the PluralPlus companion website features additional resources, such as editable worksheets, sound files, and video clips.

At the heart of the book is the understanding that accents are normal and natural, representing the wonderful linguistic diversity of our species. Unfortunately, when non-native speakers have not achieved the degree of intelligibility and naturalness required for effective communication in their target language, they may face significant barriers to personal and professional success. When clients reach out for help in overcoming these hurdles, they often turn to professionals, and SLPs are well-equipped for the task. The key is to understand that although graduate training and clinical expertise provide SLPs with a solid foundation, it is their ethical obligation to attain the additional skills and knowledge necessary to produce results with this unique clientele. Fortunately this goal is well within reach, and the hope is that this book will play a role in the future success of many SLPs and their clients.

Chapter 1, "Accents," lays a foundation by considering the nature of accents and why people have them. Although each of us has an accent, a non-native accent often presents significant challenges. Fortunately, non-native speakers who acquire a clear and natural accent can overcome these obstacles and even communicate more effectively than native speakers of their new language. SLPs are well-suited to help them achieve this goal.

Chapter 2, "Accent Modification," addresses the practicalities and efficacy of accent modification and discusses the professionals who provide it, along with their settings. It also discusses the training and skills that SLPs bring to this field. This chapter introduces the useful distinction between the segmental and suprasegmental features of phonology and provides a look at the counseling aspect of accent training.

Chapter 3, "Assessment," reviews the principles involved in determining which areas of a client's speech present the greatest barriers to communicative success. While many SLPs are uncertain about how to conduct second language phonological evaluations, the goal of this chapter is to empower them to develop their own methods by adapting the ideas and materials provided in this manual.

Chapter 4, "Segmentals Overview," looks at ways to develop clients' phonemic awareness and addresses the principles involved in working with the individual sounds of the language. There is an extensive review of techniques, such as minimal pairs, some practical ideas on promoting generalization, and an in-depth look at the process of target selection.

Chapter 5, "Suprasegmentals Overview," focuses primarily on intonation and rate, since these two features can be addressed at any stage of second language phonological acquisition and form the foundation of much of the suprasegmental training that helps clients produce natural sounding speech.

Chapter 6, "Consonants," outlines the consonant inventory of English and focuses on those which tend to be the most problematic. In keeping with the "clear and natural" approach advocated in the book, phonemes which tend to have a strong effect on intelligibility, as well as the allophones which can affect naturalness, are addressed.

Chapter 7, "Vowels," bridges the gaps between the theoretical knowledge about the English vowel system that SLPs have from their courses in phonetics and phonology, and the practical aspects of eliciting these sounds with non-native speaking clients. While it is relatively rare for SLPs to work with vowels in most other areas within our scope of practice, in accent modification it is both common and powerful.

Chapter 8, "Syllables and Stress" returns to the suprasegmentals to examine several features of English that often prove troublesome for non-native speakers. Variations in syllable structure and lexical stress in the world's languages make these aspects challenging, and clinicians often make significant gains when addressing them with clients.

Chapter 9, "Prosody," uses a narrow definition of this term to address suprasegmentals related to the rhythm and phrasing of English. This chapter also examines vowel reductions, which are key to producing natural speech, and emphasis, which is often a good starting point for work on more abstract features of intonation.

Chapter 10, "Connected Speech," discusses the elements of natural spontaneous oral communication and looks into features which are rarely addressed by SLPs in other fields, such as linking and elision. The goal is to help clients develop the ability to balance intelligibility and naturalness.

Chapter 11, "Getting Started," begins with a discussion of the next steps SLPs can take to excel in accent modification and provides resources on how to get started in private practice. There is also an in-depth section on the mechanics of a university-clinic accent modification program and some words of advice from graduate students to their peers. The chapter ends with some thoughtful words from private practitioners concerning the challenges and rewards of this incredible field.

My personal journey has unfolded in the opposite direction of most SLPs working in accent modification. I had earned an M.A. in Russian Studies and an M.A. in Teaching English to Speakers of Other Languages (TESOL) before I became an SLP. In my 26-year career teaching English to non-native speakers, I worked in six countries with clients from over 80 nations, and this experience has informed my work at San Diego State University's Accent and Communication Training (ACT) program, where I have had the pleasure of supervising many outstanding graduate clinicians. My personal connection to accent comes from my experiences as a native speaker of English and non-native speaker of Hungarian, Russian, Spanish, German, and Portuguese. In the nearly 10 years of my adult life spent living abroad and communicating in other languages, I have had a glimpse of the challenges and emotions that often go hand-in-hand with sounding different. Accents and languages are a part of my home as well; my wife, who is also a practicing SLP, is a native speaker of Hungarian, and my son is a bilingual speaker of Hungarian and English. A love of languages, accents, and cultures brought me to this field, and if it brought you here as well, I know you will be rewarded by working with this amazing group of clients.

*Dedicated to Szilvi and Mark, whose accents lie in my heart.*

# CHAPTER

# 1

# Accents

## Our Accents

We each have an accent. We overlook this universal truth because we consider our own way of speaking as normal and speech that differs as accented. In the words of Peter Ladefoged, "an accent is always what the other person has." (Ladefoged & Disner, 2012, p. 27) This is especially true if we speak the "standard" or "prestige" dialect of a language. Upon examination, this reasoning collapses quickly. It is important to understand that each one of us has an accent, and we sometimes use the word *idiolect* to highlight the fact that just as our voices are unique, so are our individual patterns of speaking. The way we speak is who we are. Native speakers are conjoined by the commonalities of their individual accents, creating a powerful sense of community. Yet for non-native speakers, a way of speaking that differs can pose significant challenges. The phonology of each language is unique, and if a non-native speaker is unable to produce particular sounds in the new language, miscommunication may result. In addition, speech produced with patterns dissimilar to a target language may cause listeners to focus on the delivery and not the message. Many non-native speakers devote time and energy to mastering the pronunciation of a target language because they believe that changing the way they speak can help them attain the personal and professional success they desire. Accent modification is an elective service that assists clients in achieving their goals, and speech-language pathologists (SLPs) are especially well-suited to provide it.

## Native Accents

Accents and attitudes about them represent incredibly complex phenomena, and the concept of a *native accent* is an important starting point in any discussion of second language phonology. The word *accent* tends to be interpreted in two different ways. Crystal (2008, p. 3) defined *accent* broadly as the "features of pronunciation which identify

1

where a person is from, regionally, and socially," but Scovel (1969, p. 38) defined accent in the narrower sense as "phonological cues, either segmental or suprasegmental, which identify the speaker as a non-native user of the language." According to the first definition, everyone has an accent, but by the second definition, some of us do and some of us do not, and this division of the world into native and non-native speakers has profound implications. Subtle differences alone can set the non-native apart even when there is no effect on communication. From a very early age, native speakers of a language are able to identify non-natives quickly, and this has a profound effect on group identity that cannot be underestimated. When non-native speakers open their mouths they can be instantaneously categorized as "other."

The word *native* is derived from the Latin verb *nāscī* stemming from the proto Indo-European root *gene-, meaning *to give birth*. Thus the use of the term "native speaker" implies that speakers born into a language will speak it differently than those who are not. The association with birth itself is imprecise; it is universally understood that humans can acquire the mother tongue they were born into and learn to sound exactly like a native speaker in a second language at a later point in life. The key question is whether this is possible throughout the lifespan or only up to a certain age. As a thought experiment, I ask my clients to imagine a 6-year-old girl from their country who is adopted by a monolingual English-speaking family and raised in the United States. When I ask whether she would have a native-sounding accent in her new language at the age of 20, they are universally certain she would. I then ask them to imagine a 20-year-old woman from their country who marries an American and moves to this country. She has some knowledge of English when she arrives and then spends 20 years speaking English to her husband, family, co-workers, and friends. When I ask my clients whether she would sound like a native or non-native by the age of 40, they generally say she will sound like a non-native, but in almost every group of clients, at least one insists she might be able to acquire a native accent. Is there evidence to support this?

This book argues that non-native accents are both natural and wonderful, and that they do not inherently interfere with communication. However, it is important to establish at the outset whether adult learners of a second language can acquire accents that sound exactly like a native speaker. This question has been the subject of considerable research and debate, but it is not an academic exercise because it has profound implications for accent modification. When non-native speakers choose to modify their accents it is common for them to aim for native-sounding speech as the ultimate level of success. Derwing (2003), asked one hundred adult second language learners in Canada to rate the degree to which they agreed with the following statement on a 7-point scale (with 7 representing "I strongly agree" and 1 representing "I strongly disagree"): "If it were possible, I would pronounce English like a native speaker." Ninety-five out of one hundred responded affirmatively, with 82% rating their agreement as a 1 and 13% selecting 2. Many books and websites promote the idea that non-natives can lose their accent as a central selling point to attract customers. In addition, many natives tend to consider any differences between a learner's speech and the native model as imperfections that should be corrected, and it is unfair to those acquiring a second language to pretend otherwise even if we could eliminate these unfortunate biases in a perfect world. If attaining a native accent as an adult can be reliably achieved, SLPs' focus should be on determining exactly how to produce that result. On the other hand, if achieving this goal is extremely rare (if not entirely impossible) then disappointment is bound to follow, and we are setting our clients up for failure. In reality, the research has shown that for those who acquire a language at some point during or after adolescence, having an accent is expected. Clients should be encouraged to understand that they are normal; it is entirely natural to have an accent. The goal of accent modification is to help our clients communicate effectively, which is something SLPs are well-trained to do, and not to make them indistinguishable from native speakers of the target language, which is unrealistic and unnecessary. Nevertheless, because it is so widely believed by non-natives and natives alike that adults can "lose" their accents, this notion merits a more detailed investigation, and it is always worth exploring with clients before training begins.

## The Critical Period

Throughout the ages, adults have envied the advantages children enjoy in learning a second language, but serious study of children's relative facility dates only to the second half of the twentieth century. Balari and Lorenzo (2015) cite Juan Huarte de San Juan, a pioneer in cognitive psychology, as stating in 1575 that, "children, as already observed by Aristotle, learn any single language better than older men, in spite of the latter being more rational. And no one needs to remember us this, for common experience amply shows it, as when a thirty or forty years old native from Biscay [Basque Country] comes to Castile, and he never learns the Romance language, but if he is a child, within two or three years he looks as if born in Toledo." The modern era of research became active by the 1960s, picked up steam in the 1990s, and continues to the present day. Penfield and Roberts (1959) linked children's second language abilities to ongoing neuroplasticity, which is subsequently diminished through maturation. Lenneberg (1967, p. 176) was the first to conclude that "foreign accents cannot be overcome easily after puberty," highlighting the uniqueness of phonology in second language acquisition and demarcating the boundaries of attainment on par with native speakers. This *critical period hypothesis* (CPH) posits a developmental point after which biological changes preclude second language learners from achieving nativelike competence in a language. Scovel (1969) attributed the inability to acquire nativelike proficiency after puberty to neuroplasticity, but others, including Patkowski (1990), sought to disassociate lateralization from plasticity. Long (1990) offered decreasing myelination during development as an alternative mechanism to explain the change in plasticity. Birdsong (2018) reports that: "more recent researchers have put forth other neurobiological explanations for plasticity deficits over age. For example, on a 'use it then lose' it model, after adolescence the circuitry that is required for language learning is dismantled because in adulthood there remains no selection pressure on humans to keep learning languages."

Several different strands of research related to CPH have emerged. Much research has focused on language acquisition in general, with a great deal of attention paid to second language acquisition, and specifically, second language phonology, because it appears to follow different acquisition patterns than other aspects of language. Many studies have attempted to define this critical period by identifying its ages of onset and offset. In other words, what is the earliest age a child might be immersed in a second language and speak with a non-native accent and what is the latest age someone can acquire a language and sound like a native? Studies have also addressed the linearity of the critical period and whether it should be defined as a *sensitive period* (SP) to avoid falsification by exceptional learners. After analyzing previous research on the issue, Long (1990, p. 274) lowered traditional estimates for the age of onset, claiming that "exposure needs to occur before age 6 to guarantee that L2 phonology can become nativelike." He based this conclusion on several long-term studies, including Oyama's (1976) examination of sixty Italian immigrants to the United States. In that study, several children with an age of arrival between six and ten were found to have an accent in English, despite lengthy periods of residence in their adopted country. While Lenneberg (1967) cited puberty as the point after which non-native speakers could not achieve accent free speech, despite the presumably wide variation at which this process occurs in individuals, Scovel (1969) specified age twelve as the age of offset, and this number has been used consistently as a benchmark in studies of second language acquisition. Long concurred that age twelve represented the upper limit of the critical period, and he identified the age of six as the age of onset. More recently, Granena and Long (2013, p. 336) reaffirmed this timeframe, stating: ". . . the evidence from this study, plus from previous research by others, leads to the conclusion that there is an SP for phonology, its offset beginning at age six, and possibly earlier . . . probably closing by age 12." It is important to note that there is no reason to believe that any specific age will ever be identified, so these timeframes are generalizations. As Munro and Mann (2005, p. 337) point out: "[no] model of an age–accent connection should ever hope to claim 'before age X, a person is guaranteed to develop a native accent and, after age Y, a foreign accent is unavoidable'" On balance, however, the preponderance of evidence indicates that most non-native speakers will speak with a foreign accent if they are immersed in a second language after about the age of twelve, although the age of offset of the sensitive period for some speakers may come a few years later. The individual variations found between these ages lend credence to the notion of a sensitive period as opposed to a critical period.

## Ultimate Attainment

The relevance of the critical period to accent modification is clear—it is natural for adults to have accents. Many factors can affect a non-native accent. Some may be within the control of the speaker, such as motivation, amount of practice, formal study of the language, and length of residence in a country where the language is spoken; others are beyond the speaker's control, such as native language or linguistic aptitude. Nevertheless, if we control for all of these factors, the most significant variable is still the age of immersion in the target language environment.

If we end the discussion by agreeing that the age at which someone is immersed in a foreign language is strongly predictive of whether that person will speak with a native or non-native accent, then we miss one crucial point that is inextricably tied to the world of accent modification: what can an adult learner ultimately attain in terms of a nativelike accent? In other words, is it ever possible for an adult learner to speak another language with a native accent? There is strong evidence suggesting that the answer is no. Despite this fact, many non-native speakers strive to sound exactly like natives and many natives expect them to do so.

It is important to analyze this issue in detail because we know that many non-native speakers cite native-sounding speech as their goal. As discussed above, Derwing (2003) quantified the percentage of learners who desired this outcome at 95%, and it is easy to understand why this number is so high. Being capable of sounding like a native implies that the speaker is still able to sound non-native as well, but the reverse is not true. Given the choice between two possible outcomes of learning a second language—one in which you could choose to sound exactly like a native whenever you liked, and another in which you would always sound non-native, which one would you choose? Intellectually, we can agree that there is no good reason for native-sounding speakers to have advantages over non-native-sounding speakers, but it would be wishful thinking to deny the tremendous amount of discrimination that occurs based solely on the way someone sounds when they speak, even if it is unrelated to issues such as intelligibility and naturalness, and it would be unreasonable to sidestep the expectations of our clients and the native speakers they interact with.

Several studies dating back to the 1990s have attempted to falsify the critical period theory with evidence of exceptional learners who attained native-sounding speech despite being late learners of a language. Ioup, Boustagui, El Tigi, and Moselle (1994), analyzed Julie, a highly successful late second language learner, who as a twenty-one-year-old monolingual British immigrant to Egypt, found herself immersed in an exclusively Arabic environment when her husband was unexpectedly called into the Egyptian military. During a 45-day period spent with her monolingual, Arabic-speaking in-laws, Julie began to acquire Arabic; within two years she was often mistaken for a native speaker. Ioup et al. collected a spontaneous speech sample by asking Julie and several native-speaking controls to talk about their favorite recipes. Julie was rated as a native speaker by 7 of the 13 judges. Other studies have also reported on exceptional learners who attained native-sounding speech as evidenced by self-ratings or native-speaker ratings of recorded phrases or spontaneous speech (Moyer, 1999; Nikolov, 2009; Piller, 2002).

In a more thorough analysis, Abrahamsson and Hyltenstam (2009) studied 195 Spanish-Swedish bilinguals who self-identified as having native Swedish accents, and found that none of the speakers who acquired Swedish after age 17 were able to pass as native speakers after rigorous examination, concluding that "absolute nativelikeness in late learners, in principle, does not occur." They argued that previous reports of exceptional learners were identified due to "subjective, and unverified observations, . . . inappropriate definitions of nativelikeness or insufficiently sophisticated techniques for linguistic scrutiny." (p. 292)

It can be difficult to evaluate evidence of exceptional learners. Anecdotal reports are often made by non-natives, who may not be able to judge native speech accurately. Second-hand reports of native speakers complimenting someone on their nativelike speech tend to be more likely due to flattery than intensive phonological analysis. Scovel (1988, p. 177) points out that in some cases, ". . . when they say, 'I'm amazed that you sound just like a native!' they are really saying something like 'You speak my language brilliantly—especially for a foreigner!'" Objective measures used in research may be insufficient due to a ceiling effect: a non-native might pass for a native when reading a sentence but not when several minutes of spontaneous speech are examined. In fact, it is essentially possible for any adult learner to pass for a native speaker depending on the conditions. A non-native may be mistaken for a native when saying a single word, reciting a prepared phrase, or speaking in a loud environment, but this is not what is generally understood to mean by acquiring a native accent. In order to bolster the argument that nativelike speech is not truly acquired by late learners, this book uses another type of evidence.

## Actors and Spies

In almost every profession, speakers who have an accent but communicate effectively can carry out their work as well as a native speaker, but there are two professions that come to mind when considering occupations in which even a trace of an accent might cause significant difficulties: acting and undercover spying. Actors work hard to create the illusion that they are someone else, so actors playing native-speaking American characters need to sound as if they were born in the United States. In a similar vein, but with higher stakes, deep cover spies or "moles" need to convince others that they are part of the very societies they are working against. By examining the role of accent in these two professions, we can find more evidence for the notion that attaining accents that are indistinguishable from native versions appears to be extremely rare, if not entirely impossible.

To shape their performances, successful actors must have, almost by definition, above average abilities to observe the voices and gestures of those around them and to mimic them accurately. When training for their roles, they are careful to create an identity for their character that will ring true for their audience. Many actors have been successful at sounding exactly like speakers of other dialects of their language when they are on the stage or screen. Hugh Laurie, who is originally from England and normally speaks with a British accent, played an American character successfully for eight seasons on the television series *House*, and many Americans reported that they only realized he was not from the United States when they heard him speaking in his native dialect during interviews. British actors have a strong tradition of voice training, and television and movies expose them to a great deal of American English, but actors from around the world also appear to be able to imitate mutually intelligible dialects when reading their lines.

The key points above are "performance" and "dialect." Hugh Laurie practiced his dialog carefully before each episode, and even then reported that he dreaded certain words or phrases such as *New York* because he felt he could never say them with credible rhoticity (Rose, 2012). Although he could probably get through a day speaking American

English without anyone realizing his origins, it would not be easy. This is an important point to keep in mind because the actual incidence of natives acquiring a second dialect to the point where they blend into their new environment completely is considered to be very low (Siegel, 2012). Moreover, when it comes to languages, as opposed to dialects, actors have an entirely different track record. Meryl Streep is frequently lauded for her skill with accents, but this is generally in reference to either her ability to accurately produce a dialect of English or English spoken with a non-native accent. When actors with considerable imitation skills play roles in which they must speak a foreign language as a native, they are virtually always identifiable as having an accent by speakers of that language. Robin Williams, an incredibly talented mimic, studied Russian for five hours a day for five months before undertaking his role of a Muscovite in *Moscow on the Hudson* (Blau, 1984), and he performed much of the movie's dialog in that language with an impressive accent that nevertheless, would not convince a Russian audience that he was born there. Meryl Streep also worked meticulously to develop her accent for the lines she delivered in Polish in the movie *Sophie's Choice* (Maslin, 1982), but Poles, while impressed with her effort, would not mistake her for a native. There have been many stars and supporting players who learned English as adults and found success in Hollywood, but they are not cast in roles that require the audience to believe they are native speakers. When they are cast in such roles, audiences may notice and the suspension of belief evaporates. There are exceptions, such as Christoph Waltz, the gifted multilingual actor from Vienna, who played an American character in the movie *Big Eyes*, but directors understand that this is a gamble because the audience will likely notice that the actor is not a native speaker. It is also noteworthy that in virtually every case in which an actor or actress has portrayed a native speaker of English without having had significant pre-pubescent exposure to the language, their native language has been from the Germanic branch of the Indo-European language family, and typically a close relative of English, such as Dutch. In short, given the level of talent and motivation of the non-native English-speaking actors around the globe, the fact that none of them routinely play native-speaking Americans serves as anecdotal evidence of how difficult this is to achieve.

Similarly, in the world of espionage, intelligence agencies from around the world have high motivation to train their agents to infiltrate another country by speaking its language in a way that would not draw attention. The notion of deep cover spies who are trained to speak another language perfectly has been popularized by spy novels and movies, but the reality is quite different. In the former Soviet Union, a 1970s television mini-series, *Seventeen Moments of Spring*, captured the nation's attention by portraying the exploits of a Russian intelligence officer who was able to infiltrate the Nazi high command in the closing days of World War II. The series is said to be based on the real-life exploits of Nikolai Kuznetsov, who was born near the Urals but could pass for German even though he had never traveled outside of his home country. It is difficult to assess his actual abilities since he died in the war and was lionized immediately afterward, but it is important to note two relevant points. First, his interactions with Germans were relatively short, and second, he was careful to never speak the particular German dialect of his interlocutors, so as an analogy, if he had operated in English he might have chosen an

Irish dialect when talking to someone from New York. Despite his apparent success, this type of case is extremely rare; in the history of espionage, virtually all undercover spies had significant pre-pubescent exposure to their target language, whether by birth in an environment where the language is spoken or from interaction with a native-speaking parent.

Several recent spy stories attest to this phenomenon. Jack Barsky was an East German spy recruited by the KGB to penetrate West Germany in the 1970s. During his training in Moscow it was discovered that he had an incredible talent for accent and had acquired English exceptionally quickly. The KGB decided to take a risk and send him to work as a sleeper agent in the United States, where he would attempt to pass himself off as an American with a German mother. Although he was never activated, he was caught by the FBI, but because he had never actually spied and was able to provide useful information, he was never charged with a crime and went on to become a U.S. citizen and author. This story provides several important insights. First, his accent abilities predated his training to become a sleeper agent. In other words, the KGB did not train him to speak with a nearly flawless native accent, but rather they exploited his unique gift. Second, the fact that he was given a cover story of having a German mother indicates his handlers were nervous that someone might pick up on traces of his accent.

The FX channel series, *The Americans*, depicts a group of Soviet agents trained to blend into American society, and it bears a loose resemblance to actual events that unfolded in 2010 as the FBI arrested 10 Russian agents who had moved into an American neighborhood to create a spy base. When events like this reach the public's attention, they feed into the belief that spies can achieve native-sounding accents. On a website devoted to a language teaching business promising fluency in just 3 months, the owner refers to this specific group of spies and argues that they had achieved accents that were indistinguishable from native speakers, with the implication that others could do the same with the right techniques and effort. In fact, even though some of these agents spoke excellent English, they generally pretended to be from Belgium or Quebec since it was obvious to any casual listener that they were not native speakers. The agent with the accent closest to native (Andrei Bezrukov) has given many interviews in English, and his slight accent is easily detectable within seconds. Thus, even when a sophisticated foreign intelligence service attempts to plant non-native speakers into another society, their trained agents cannot truly pass for natives, and a search of the annals of world espionage provides no counterevidence.

In the final analysis, non-native speakers who are proficient in English and have intelligible and natural pronunciation can do well in any job they choose, and accent should not be a barrier. The two notable exceptions are spying and acting, and for those professions the accent itself can determine success. While the public holds onto the belief that spies, actors, and other non-native speakers often break the odds and achieve nativelike accents, a critical review of the scientific evidence and historical record disproves this claim.

Perhaps you know someone who has learned a language without significant exposure to it in their youth and can speak it without sounding any different than a native. These exceptional learners may exist, but if so, they are exceedingly rare. Perhaps more importantly for those of us working in the field of accent modification, we do not know how they got there, and it certainly was not because of our work. Derwing and Munro (2015, p. 34), who have spent decades researching accents, state unequivocally, "no study has ever shown that instruction or other systematic training can help adult L2 learners to speak with a perfectly nativelike accent at all times under all conditions." On the other hand, we can all cite many examples of non-native language learners who achieve nativelike phonological proficiency, although they are still identifiable as non-natives. This is a practical and achievable outcome for anyone, and accent modification can play a significant role in bringing it about.

# Effective Communication

While some clients may have difficulty accepting the permanence of their accents, it is important to let them know that the accent itself does not have to be the source of their miscommunications. Clients should be proud of their backgrounds and the hard work they put into mastering another tongue. Their accents may set them apart, but they should not interfere significantly with the personal or professional success of non-native speakers if they are effective communicators. There are successful non-natives in virtually every profession in the world. For example, we encounter successful non-native speech-language pathologists, lawyers, teachers, doctors, air-traffic controllers, homemakers, and counselors.

A good analogy to highlight the shift away from focusing on eliminating traces of a non-native accent is the nature of dialects that bear similarities to one another. Languages have regional and social dialects, and in most cases, differences in speaking do not interfere with intelligibility or naturalness. When a speaker of American English communicates with someone from Ireland, for example, there is no doubt in either speaker's mind that they grew up speaking different versions of English, yet they have little difficulty exchanging complex thoughts efficiently. Each speaker may spend some extra time processing language when segmentals or suprasegmentals stray from their expected targets, but there is minimal effect on overall communication. Speakers from Ireland do not need to sound exactly like speakers of American English to achieve their personal or professional goals in the United States, nor would Americans need to adopt an Irish dialect to succeed in the Republic of Ireland. In much the same way, non-native speakers may have accents that mark them as coming from a different part of the world, but they are capable of being equal and even better communicators in English than their native-speaking peers.

As another analogy, beyond the world of language, think of speakers of each language of the world as playing both a different instrument and a different style of music. We might imagine a speaker of English playing violin and a speaker of Mandarin Chinese playing piano. In order to make music successfully in the American style, the Chinese musician does not have to concentrate on making the piano sound just like a violin. Instead, the goal is to adapt to the new musical style. The instruments will sound different, but the music they make together can be beautiful.

## Accentedness

Intuitively, we understand that accents are patterns of speech that we use to identify which speakers belong to a certain group and which ones do not. The group can expand or contract depending on who is in the comparison group. A speaker of an English dialect typical of Boston might identify a speaker from New York as having a different accent, but once a speaker from London walks in the room, the Bostonian and New Yorker may both identify themselves as speakers of American English. If a speaker from Germany walks in the room, the three native English speakers may now form a new group in contrast to the lone non-native. Humans are remarkably adept at identifying accents from an early age, even in infancy (Nazzi, Jusczyk, & Johnson, 2000) and even after hearing a mere 30 ms of speech (Flege, 1984), yet a precise linguistic definition of the term eludes us. As Lippi-Green (2012) points out in her book *English with an Accent*, ". . . in so far as linguists are concerned, the term *accent* has no technical or specific meaning." One point of clarification we can add is that the term *accent* traditionally excludes differences in vocabulary and grammar, so any operational definition will be centered on the segmental and supra-segmental elements of speech.

For our purposes, the fact that humans know an accent when they hear one means we do not need an exact definition of the term. We will define accent as those recognizable elements of speech that allow us to sort speakers into meaningful groups, and because acquiring a native accent continues to be the goal of so many adults learning a second language, we will generally be considering native versus non-native accents. In order to highlight a distinction between variations in speech that have a negative impact on communication from those that do not, we can use the term *accentedness*. This is neither a precise nor objective term, but it is useful in helping us identify appropriate targets for accent modification. The importance of using this term is that it allows us to separate mere variation from differences that affect the ability to convey information. In fact, many people conflate these two ideas, and that often serves to fuel the desire to "eliminate" an accent. In pioneering work, Munro and Derwing (1995) found that accentedness, intelligibility, and comprehensibility (which will be examined in more detail below) were not perfectly correlated. In other words, while speakers who showed signs of being difficult to understand were generally rated by native-speaking listeners as having a strong accent, some speakers who were considered to have strong accents were 100% intelligible. This groundbreaking study drove a wedge between the concepts of nativeness (i.e., sounding exactly like a native speaker) and intelligibility.

Since we have good evidence that native accents are rare if not impossible to acquire in adulthood, and we also know they are not essential to convey ideas accurately in a second language, we can guide clients to an understanding that the goal of accent modification is to improve communication—not to pass for a native speaker. Miscommunications are a part of life for everyone, but when non-natives have significantly more miscommunications than natives, they often take steps to address the issue. Accent work focuses on helping non-natives become effective communicators, and this is a realistic and achievable goal.

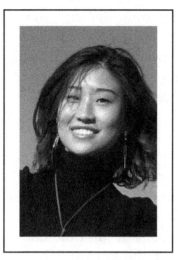

Accents do not make non-native speakers inferior to native speakers. Having an accent is normal and there is nothing wrong about it. Accents do not define whether a person is intelligent or not, though it reveals where one is from. In addition, accents actually increase the diversity of language. As long as one can be understood, one's accent isn't a problem in communication.

—Yiyang Shen, Accent Modification Client

There are countless non-natives throughout the world who are better communicators in comparison to their peers who speak with native accents. Thus, sharing ideas efficiently is the overarching goal clients need to embrace.

## Nativeness Versus Intelligibility

This pedagogical debate concerning the appropriateness of focusing on acquiring a perfect native accent versus focusing on being understood is not new in the study of second language phonological acquisition, and it is typically labeled *nativeness versus intelligibility*. Arguments against focusing on nativeness have come from a variety of directions aside from those outlined above. Some feel that a bias (often implicit) toward nativeness as the ultimate level of attainment is a form of linguistic imperialism. Non-native speakers often face a great deal of bias and prejudice based on the way they speak, and by subtly implying that their accents in and of themselves are inferior, we become at best bystanders to this discrimination, and at worst, promoters of it. Others have suggested that because English has become a lingua franca, there is no need to choose one particular form of English pronunciation as a model. While these arguments have merit, most non-natives still prefer to acquire an accent indistinguishable from the majority of their everyday interlocutors (Derwing, 2003). The most effective argument against nativeness is perhaps that it is both extremely elusive and demonstrably less important than other factors. When we take nativeness off the table, we are frequently left with the proposed alternative of intelligibility. This makes sense because intelligibility lies at the very heart of communication, and it has been studied since the earliest days of speech science. Communication involves sharing ideas, and if a client is not intelligible, thoughts are not perceived accurately. On an intuitive level, we understand that when we say that someone has a good accent, the underlying implication is that intelligibility is very high. It would be unusual to hear someone say, "She has a great accent. I don't understand anything she says, but it's a great accent!" When native speakers communicate, they have near 100% intelligibility in most cases, and this is certainly an important goal for non-native speakers to achieve. The question becomes whether intelligibility alone guarantees effective communication, but before addressing that issue, we need to examine intelligibility in more detail.

## Intelligibility and Comprehensibility

Like the term *accent*, the concept of intelligibility is not a new one, but it has been defined in a number of different ways that share the underlying notion of accurate recognition of speech. It has also taken on a greater significance in our era of electronic communication. All oral communication by humans occurred literally within earshot until the mid-19th century, but now we have the capability to convey speech between the earth and the moon, as well as from this moment to the distant future, and this has involved huge technological advances dependent on accurate transmission of spoken words. Pickering (2006, p. 220) points out that "there is no universally agreed upon definition of what constitutes this construct, nor is there an agreed upon way of measuring it," but the core idea is simple enough: intelligibility is the amount of speech that is understood. In its narrowest sense it can refer to the accurate transcription of speech at the phonemic level even when the underlying message may be entirely misconstrued, but in its broadest sense, it suggests accurate speech production, leading to a successful transmission of a message to a listener. It tends to be looked at as an objective measure, distinguished by contrasting it with other terms such as *comprehensibility* (a more subjective rating related to the listener's understanding of the message) and *interpretability* which focuses on the speaker's intentions (see Smith & Nelson, 1985). While the term *interpretability* has fallen out of favor (Levis, 2005), comprehensibility has played a large role in many recent studies of second language phonology.

Although there are also many ways to define *comprehensibility*, and there are problems related to the term because of its potential to be interpreted synonymously with *intelligibility*, Derwing and Munro's (2015, p. 3) definition is perhaps the most useful because of the importance of their work on accent research. They define *comprehensibility* as a subjective measure of "the amount of effort that must be put in to understanding speech." In their studies, Derwing and Munro have frequently contrasted objective measures, such as native-speaker transcription of non-native speech samples, or accurate responses to true/false questions, to subjective measures such as rating scales designed to peer into the amount of effort required of listeners to process speech. This distinction allows them to delineate the partially independent variables of accentedness, intelligibility (accurate transmission), and comprehensibility (listener effort).

## A Clear and Natural Accent

If effective communication is a more appropriate objective than a native accent, is focusing on intelligibility and comprehensibility the best way to achieve it? The case for intelligibility is strong; speakers need to be understood in order to share their thoughts. Moreover, given our training and experience it is natural for SLPs to place a heavy emphasis on intelligibility. SLPs tend to have backgrounds working on articulation with children who are native speakers, and in these cases they work on improving their clients' ability to produce phonemes accurately. This segmental approach is effective because children with articulation delays do not normally have difficulties with suprasegmental aspects of speech unrelated to the difficulties they have with specific sounds. In other words, SLPs do not generally have to address aspects such as intonation, phrasing, linking, and stress; they simply need to elicit accurate production of specific sounds. Unfortunately, when working with non-native speakers, that approach may overlook other important elements of communication.

Clients seek accent modification for a variety of reasons, but the prime motivation is often a desire to be understood. However, intelligibility is not the only goal clients need to have. If we consider intelligibility to mean the percentage of a speaker's utterances that can be accurately transcribed, then we would have to consider the case of a non-native speaker who produces highly intelligible speech that has plodding or unnatural prosody. Here, the speaker's message can be conveyed accurately, but because the way it is produced is so unnatural, listeners will spend time and energy focusing on how the speaker is talking instead of what was said. Therefore, non-native speakers need to produce the patterns of English in a way that is similar enough to the way native speakers produce them; it is not enough to simply be understood.

SLPs work with an amazing range of communication difficulties aside from articulation, and some of these other areas offer insight into the need to move past a focus on intelligibility (and even comprehensibility). One example comes from experiences working with children with autism spectrum disorders. Many times, speech-related communication difficulties with these clients are completely unrelated to intelligibility or comprehensibility. Imagine speech produced in a monotone with the intermittent interjection of a catchphrase by a speaker using minimal eye contact. The intelligibility is not compromised, and while the interjections may affect comprehensibility, the most significant impact of this type of speech is that the unusual nature of the speech causes listeners to concentrate disproportionately on how the child is speaking, as opposed to what the child is saying.

Consider also experiences with clients who stutter. A person whose stutter is characterized by moderate prolongations and repetitions will not generally face challenges regarding intelligibility. Comprehensibility may be compromised because extra effort is required to understand the speaker, but more importantly listeners become uncomfortable and may complete the speaker's sentences or make unwarranted judgments, and this is more likely due to the lack of naturalness.

As SLPs, we know communication can be divided between what someone says and how they say it, and this division is an especially effective way of looking at the communicative effectiveness of non-native speakers. Above all, non-native speakers must be as close to 100% intelligible as possible, and when working with clients I usually call this being *clear*, but they must also adhere to the general patterns of native speech and pragmatics, and I call this being *natural*. Naturalness has been used as a measure for several aspects of speech, including fluency (Langevin, Kully, Teshima, Hagler, Narasimha, &

Prasad, 2010), dysarthria (Anand & Stepp, 2015), and alaryngeal speech (Eadie & Doyle, 2003). In fact, Anand and Stepp's (2015, p. 1135) definition of naturalness seems to fit perfectly into our work with second language phonological acquisition. They considered speech to be natural "if it conforms to the listener's standards of rate, rhythm, intonation, stress patterning, and if it conforms to the syntactic structure of the utterance being produced."

In this modified paradigm, we can view *accentedness* as what marks someone as a speaker of another language, independent of any impact on communicative effectiveness, *intelligibility* as the ability to be understood, and *naturalness* as the amount listeners are able to focus on what is being said versus how it is said.

This "clear and natural" approach, may take some practice for many SLPs who are accustomed to focusing primarily on segmentals and who have backgrounds helping children produce highly accurate speech. It is often natural for SLPs to counsel non-natives to speak slowly or use extremely clear enunciation, but the end result is that they may sound less fluent, which diminishes the effectiveness of their communication. Fortunately, SLPs can apply their expertise in working on all of the multifaceted aspects of communication and can rely on their training and experiences working with clients facing a variety of communicative challenges.

Many accent trainers and SLPs (as well as some clients) may resist the idea of natural speech because they consider these more spontaneous forms to be inferior to clearly enunciated speech. There is generally a bias in favor of clear and careful speech independent of the communicative context, but the goal should be to give clients the ability to note how different registers co-exist and to understand when and how to use them. Generally, clients underestimate how common natural speech is in comparison to careful speech, but as they encounter native speakers in their personal and professional lives, this awareness develops and they begin to increase the naturalness of their own communication.

## Awareness, Training, and Counseling

There is a great deal of mystery surrounding accents. When people begin to study a foreign language, they may assume that pronunciation will come easily or that it will be relatively trivial to master in comparison to grammar and vocabulary. When they continue to be recognized as someone with an accent, they may assume that they have done something wrong or have not invested enough effort in mastering the language. Native speakers may hold similar misconceptions and may judge non-natives harshly based on the way they speak, even when they have never acquired a second language themselves. Raising awareness is a wonderful way of lifting this fog and helping non-natives concentrate on overcoming communication challenges related to intelligibility and naturalness. Many clients are visibly relieved to learn that accents are normal and natural, and that becoming a more effective communicator is an achievable goal. When SLPs train clients to produce the sounds and patterns of English clearly and naturally, a focus on building awareness is crucial. Much of the change that occurs will take considerable practice on the part of the client, but developing an awareness of how English works and how it differs from their native language is often the spark that leads to success.

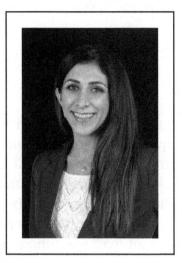

I moved to the U.S. at the age of 20 and starting a new life required speaking English as a second language. Even though learning a new language brings a new identity and culture, and it is a way to express that "we're the same," an accent barrier can translate to "we're different." In addition, people express their excitement when they meet you, but the first question they ask is, "Where are you from?" and sometimes based on the answer, there will be judgment. If you've never experienced learning another language and you meet someone who has a pronounced accent when they speak English, the fact that they can't speak like you reinforces your judgment. Maybe you feel they are less intelligent, less trustworthy, or less educated. However, if the person who doesn't look like you speaks English fluently with no accent, you will have a different perspective. Having an accent can have a significant impact on your career and social life.

—Afsaneh Ezzatyar, Accent Modification Client

While awareness is key to changes in behavior, SLPs can use their skills to train clients directly on their speech production to good effect. In many ways, this is the most natural component of accent modification for an SLP because of our experience working directly with clients. We prefer the term *training* in the field of accent modification in recognition of the fact that our clients do not have any disorders to treat; rather, they are choosing to modify their speech to communicate more effectively.

Finally, we need to consider the counseling element involved in accent modification. Speakers who are misunderstood or frequently asked to repeat themselves may shy away from others or avoid speaking. They may harbor shame and feel that they are less worthy than their native-speaking peers. They may have difficulties forming friendships or beginning relationships with native speakers, which can impact their ability to assimilate in a society. At work, they can be passed over for promotions or face subtle, or even open, discrimination. They may even be mocked or ridiculed because of the way they speak. Because of the difficulties faced by non-native speakers, those working with clients on accent modification need to be prepared to offer counseling and coaching as a part of their services. As a part of counseling clients, it is important to set realistic goals. Most clients seeking accent modification services are highly motivated, but they may have unrealistic expectations about losing their accent. It is unethical to promise attainment of a native accent when such an outcome is extremely rare. A more honest approach is to counsel that accents are normal and expected, but to also let clients know that their concerns about discrimination and difficulties are justified. Listen carefully when they discuss challenges they face but guide them to an understanding that, in most cases, they are not a result of the accent per se, but are instead due to some other aspects of their speech that can be improved with awareness and practice. Clients feel empowered when they understand that the goal is effective communication, and that they can indeed be equal or better communicators than native speakers.

## Our Role

SLPs work predominantly with people who have communicative disorders. When we study childhood language acquisition, we learn that each language has norms for when children will acquire the sounds of the language. Although there are some commonalities across languages for when children acquire the sounds of the language, each language has different norms because the phonemic inventories and relative frequencies of individual phonemes differ across languages. In the realm of L2 acquisition after puberty, norms do not exist. We expect everyone on the planet to acquire at least one language, and when there are difficulties or delays in this process, we call it a disorder and attempt to intervene. When someone learns another language as an adult, there are no expectations. We know that many people make an effort to learn another language with widely varying results. Some adults can move to another country and pick up the language relatively quickly, while others cannot master the language after decades.

Learning a second language as an adult generally requires a great deal of effort, and even after a substantial commitment of time and energy, non-native speakers may struggle to communicate in their new language. When an accent causes miscommunications or draws disproportionate attention, non-native speakers can face significant consequences

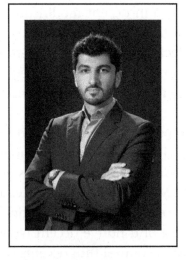

Having a foreign accent made me feel self-conscious. Even though accent modification specialists said my accent is not strong and that it would require advanced and tailored training, perhaps the hardest part is that people often shut off after the first sentence or they tell themselves they need to wait and hear it again and this time listen more carefully to understand because of the accent. When meeting new people, they rush to ask where I'm from or whether I'm visiting even though I have been in the states for the past ten years! An accent is considered appealing and it means you likely speak other language(s). However, when often the first reply in a conversation is "Excuse me," or "I didn't get that," you are not on a very good start for open and fluid communication.

—Hamzeh Omari, Accent Modification Client

in their personal and professional lives, ranging from open discrimination and hostility to subtle implicit bias.

SLPs are communication experts, and it is a natural fit for us to work with clients on accent modification. The American Speech-Language-Hearing Association (ASHA) lists accent twice in its 2016 Scope of Practice in Speech-Language Pathology—first under its list of "prevention and wellness programs," which includes the areas of practice traditionally associated with our field, and again under a shorter list of elective services, which includes professional voice use and transgender communication. The training SLPs receive gives them many advantages when working with non-native speech, but it is also important to be open to ideas that come from other fields and to spend some time becoming familiar with the aspects of accent modification that make it unique. While some SLPs take the plunge and work on accent modification full time, others use their knowledge and experience as a resource for the non-native speakers they encounter in their personal and professional lives. Just as we have much to offer non-natives who hope to become better communicators, working with non-native speakers opens the doors to a world of language and culture that enriches our lives as well.

# References

Abrahamsson, N., & Hyltenstam, K. (2009). Age of onset and nativelikeness in a second language: Listener perception versus linguistic scrutiny. *Language Learning, 59*(2), 249–306.

American Speech-Language-Hearing Association. (2016). Scope of Practice in Speech-Language Pathology. Retrieved from http://www.asha.org/policy

Anand, S., & Stepp, C. (2015). Listener perception of monopitch, naturalness, and intelligibility for speakers with Parkinson's disease. *Journal of Speech, Language, and Hearing Research, 58* (4), 1134–1144.

Balari, S., & Lorenzo, G. (2015) Should it stay or should it go? A critical reflection on the critical period for language. *Biolinguistics, 9*, 8–42.

Birdsong, D. (2018). Plasticity, variability and age in second language acquisition and bilingualism. *Frontiers in Psychology, 9*, 81. http://doi.org/10.3389/fpsyg.2018.00081

Blau, E. (1984). The ethnic authenticity of Moscow. *New York Times.* Retrieved from https://www.nytimes.com/1984/05/22/movies/the-ethnic-authenticity-of-moscow.html

Crystal, D. (2008). *A dictionary of linguistics and phonetics.* Oxford, UK: Blackwell Publishing.

Derwing, T. M., & Munro, M. J. (1997). Accent, intelligibility, and comprehensibility: Evidence from four L1s. *Studies in Second Language Acquisition, 19*, 1–16.

Derwing, T. (2003). What do ESL students say about their accents? *Canadian Modern Language Review, 59*(4), 547–566.

Derwing, T., & Munro, M. (2015). *Pronunciation fundamentals: Evidence-based perspectives for L2 teaching and research.* Philadelphia, PA: John Benjamins Publishing Company.

Eadie, T., & Doyle, P. (2003). Direct magnitude estimation and interval scaling of naturalness and severity in tracheoesophageal (TE) speakers. *Journal of Speech, Language, and Hearing Research, 45*, 1088–1096.

Flege, J. E. (1984). The detection of French accent by American listeners. *Journal of the Acoustical Society of America, 76*, 692–707.

Granena, G., & Long, M. (2013). Age of onset, length of residence, language aptitude, and ultimate L2 attainment in three linguistic domains. *Second Language Research, 29*(3), 311–343.

Ioup, G., Boustagui, E., El Tigi, M., & Moselle, M., (1994). A case study of successful adult SLA in a naturalistic environment. *Studies in Second Language Acquisition, 16*, 73–98.

Ladefoged, P., & Disner, S. F. (2012). *Vowels and consonants*. Malden, MA: Wiley-Blackwell.

Langevin, M., Kully, D., Teshima, S., Hagler, P., Narasimha, G., & Prasad, N. (2010). Five-year longitudinal treatment outcomes of the ISTAR comprehensive stuttering program. *Journal of Fluency Disorders, 35*, 123–140.

Lenneberg, E. (1967). *Biological foundations of language*. New York, NY: Wiley.

Levis, J. (2005). Changing contexts and shifting paradigms in pronunciation teaching. *TESOL Quarterly, 39*, 369–377.

Lippi-Green, R. (2012). *English with an accent: Language, ideology, and discrimination in the United States*. London and New York, NY: Routledge.

Long, M. (1990). Maturational constraints on language development. *Studies in Second Language Acquisition, 12*, 251–285.

Maslin, J. (1982). Bringing 'Sophie's Choice' to the Screen. New York Times. Retrieved from https://www.nytimes.com/1982/05/09/movies/bringing-sophie-s-choice-to-the-screen.html

Moyer, A. (1999). Ultimate attainment in L2 phonology. *Studies in Second Language Acquisition, 21*, 81–108.

Munro, M. J., & Derwing, T. M. (1995). Foreign accent, comprehensibility, and intelligibility in the speech of second language learners. *Language Learning, 45*, 73–97.

Munro, M., & Mann, V. (2005). Age of immersion as a predictor of foreign accent. *Applied Psycholinguistics, 26*, 311–341.

Nazzi, T., Jusczyk, P. W., & Johnson, E. K. (2000). Language discrimination by English learning 5-month-olds: Effect of rhythm and familiarity. *Journal of Memory and Language, 43*, 1–19.

Nikolov, M. (2009). The critical period hypothesis reconsidered: Successful adult learners of Hungarian and English. *International Review of Applied Linguistics in Language Teaching, 38*(2), 109–124.

Oyama, S. (1976). A sensitive period for the acquisition of a nonnative phonological system. *Journal of Psycholinguistic Research, 5*, 261–285.

Patkowski, M. (1990). Age and accent in a second language: A reply to James Emil Flege. *Applied Linguistics 11*, 73–89.

Pennfield, W., & Roberts, L. (1959). *Speech and brain mechanisms*. Princeton, NJ: Princeton University Press.

Pickering, L. (2006). Current research on intelligibility in English as a Lingua Franca. *Annual Review of Applied Linguistics, 26*, 219–233.

Piller, I. (2002). Passing for a native speaker: Identity and success in second language learning. *Journal of Sociolinguistics, 6*(2), 179–208.

Rose, L. (2012). 'House' Star Hugh Laurie and Creator David Shore on Its 8-Season Run: 'Feel Sorry For the Two of Us' *Hollywood Reporter*. Retrieved from https://www.hollywoodreporter.com/news/house-hugh-laurie-david-shore-326302

Scovel, T. (1969). Foreign accents, language acquisition, and cerebral dominance. *Language Learning, 19*, 245–253.

Scovel, T. (1988). A time to speak: A psycholinguistic inquiry into the critical period for human speech. *Studies in Second Language Acquisition, 12*(1), 84–85. doi.org/10.1017/S0272263100008779

Siegel, J. (2012). *Second dialect acquisition*. Cambridge, UK: Cambridge University Press.

Smith, L., & Nelson, C. (1985). International intelligibility of English: Directions and resources. *World Englishes, 4*, 333–342.

# 2

# Accent Modification

We know it is normal and natural to have an accent, but it is also clear that acquiring the phonology of a second language presents challenges and can result in communication problems significant enough to impose barriers to success. Many non-native speakers look to accent modification to help them overcome these obstacles. This chapter provides answers to several questions about accent modification related to who provides it, what it entails, and whether it produces results.

## Who Provides Accent Modification?

Since having an accent represents a difference and not a disorder, accent modification can be provided by members of any number of professions, but as a practical matter, most work in this field is carried out by teachers of English to speakers of other languages, SLPs, and voice and speech trainers.

### Teachers of English to Speakers of Other Languages

The vast majority of professionals working on accent modification come from the field of language teaching. When individuals learn a language in a classroom setting, they must master its grammar and vocabulary, and this generally includes work on speaking, listening, reading, and writing. At the early stages of language learning, there is usually an explicit focus on the sound system of the new language, and then as students progress, pronunciation is integrated into lessons at every level. When students are working on listening and speaking, they are usually given oral models of words, and their teachers will at times give feedback on productions. Thus, language teachers often find themselves on the front lines of accent modification since they are working with students at each phase of acquisition. In some language courses, there may be a lesson devoted entirely to pronunciation work. Typically, pronunciation is also integrated into classes that focus on speaking or oral presentation skills, and there are also programs throughout the world that offer stand-alone accent training courses (such as the Advanced Pronunciation and Fluency course I taught at UCSD Extension for 17 years), but these tend to be rare. If we consider how many providers are paid to work with clients on their English pronunciation, then the percentage who work in TESOL (Teaching English to Speakers of Other Languages) settings is unmatched, whether in English-speaking countries or abroad. Incidentally, while this book primarily uses the acronym TESOL as an umbrella term, other essentially synonymous terminology is common. ESL (English as a second language), TEFL (teaching English as a foreign language), ELT (English language teaching), and ELD (English language development) are all terms that are widely used. TESOL International Association (http://www.tesol.org/) is the name of the world's largest professional organization dedicated to teachers in that field.

There is a wide range of settings where TESOL instruction takes place. Many non-natives learn English in school starting at an early age. English is an international language and the lingua franca in many important fields, and it is no surprise that it is the most commonly learned foreign language throughout the world. Of the world's languages, English is ranked third in terms of native speakers with about 380 million, but if we add the approximately 750 million non-native speakers to the list, English reaches the number one spot for total speakers. Non-natives represent almost double the number of natives, and no other language comes close to matching this ratio. The practicality of English is undeniable; if an extraterrestrial were given the option to learn any of Earth's languages before being randomly placed anywhere on the globe, there is little doubt that English would be the safest bet to ensure the highest chance for successful communication. There are cases where refugees are forced to learn English out of necessity, and schoolchildren may have no choice in the matter, but the vast majority of adults learn English because they understand its value for them, both personally and professionally. English is widely taught at universities around the globe, and in some countries where English is not an official language, it is nevertheless the language of instruction in many classes in higher education. In addition, there are many programs in English-speaking countries for immigrants and for those wishing to acquire the language in a native setting. Schools of all sizes operate throughout the world, and English instruction is also provided by missionaries and volunteers. Many professionals provide one-on-one tutoring. Lastly, a great deal of informal (and unpaid) TESOL instruction takes place during everyday interactions between English speakers of varying proficiency levels as well.

The amount of training TESOL providers receive varies widely. At some programs, an MA in Applied Linguistics might be the entry level qualification for all instructors, but this is usually the exception to the rule. The bulk of TESOL instructors working in non-English-speaking countries are not native speakers of English, and in some countries and programs, oral proficiency is valued at a much lower level than grammar and vocabulary. In most private language schools in the United States and in most school systems throughout the world, the majority of instructors have a college degree, although it may be in an unrelated field. In some private language programs abroad, a native speaker of English may be hired without a college degree, but this is not common. In short, the field of TESOL is much less regulated than that of speech-language pathology, and the amount of training varies much more than for speech-language pathology.

Many TESOL teachers come to the field with a college degree and then attend a training program to earn a TEFL certificate. These programs tend to take anywhere from one to six months to complete and are taught throughout the world as well as online. Although the programs focus on pedagogy and best practices in instruction, for native speakers they often offer the first opportunity to reflect on how their native language works. TESOL instructors who attend these types of programs generally receive some training in pronunciation, but it might be cursory. Prior to earning my MA in TESOL, I attended my first TESOL teacher training program in the early 1990s at the International House in Budapest, where we had some exposure to the International Phonetic Alphabet (IPA) and a review of the most important suprasegmental features of English. Many years later I taught Best Methods in Teaching Pronunciation and Fluency, which is one of the required courses for the 6-month TEFL certificate program at UCSD's English Language Institute. This was a 27-hour course with both native and non-native speakers of English as students, that was designed to focus on the features of American English pronunciation and methods for teaching it. Most of the students were either current TESOL instructors in their home countries or prospective TESOL teachers, and over the years there were even a handful of SLPs looking for more training in accent modification. When I earned a master's degree in TESOL, as a part of the program there was one course dedicated entirely to oral proficiency, which addressed aspects of pronunciation and pedagogy related to teaching speaking skills. Instructors with an MA in TESOL or Applied Linguistics are expected to have good basic familiarity with broad transcription and an understanding of the segmentals and suprasegmentals of English.

While most TESOL teachers receive some training in pronunciation, a large number report that they lack the necessary training to teach it. John Murphy (2014, p. 78) reviewed 18 studies directly related to TESOL instructors' preparation to teach pronunciation and found the following five most common themes: "(1) ESL/EFL teachers feel underprepared to teach pronunciation, (2) they believe that more training in this area is needed, (3) too few teacher development programs offer a full course dedicated to pronunciation teaching, (4) more fully developed TESOL program curricula are needed for teachers to feel adequately supported by the programs in which they teach, and (5) teacher preparation programs are faulted for lacking a pedagogical focus in whatever might be the phonology-related courses they offer." The end result is that teachers often train themselves if they are assigned to teach a pronunciation course or if they wish to specialize in that area. In contrast to students who enter graduate programs to become SLPs, it is generally rare for TESOL instructors to have taken a phonetics course in college, thus their initial background knowledge is often limited. When pronunciation questions arise in classes devoted to teaching other aspects of English, such as vocabulary, listening, or grammar, instruction typically consists of modeling and possibly a minimal level of feedback. In most cases throughout the world, non-natives receive the majority of their English language instruction from non-native teachers. Although there is good evidence indicating that non-native speakers can provide highly effective accent modification, most studies looked at non-natives with high oral proficiency, and many non-native TESOL teachers may have not attained a high level of phonological proficiency despite their strengths in other areas. It is also fair to say that TESOL instructors who are natives have the advantage of being able to provide accurate models even if they lack pronunciation training, compared to non-native teachers who have not mastered English phonology.

As in the field of speech-language pathology, many TESOL instructors become special-ists in accent modification, and they may even take advantage of trainings offered to SLPs to sharpen their skills. The ability of TESOL accent specialists to produce effective results should not be underestimated as many are masters of their craft. In my professional experience, I have worked alongside TESOL instructors with absolutely no training from our field, who can easily hold their own, if not surpass, SLPs working in accent modifica-tion. In fact, while those in our field might be taken aback, some researchers have even criticized the training and methods of SLPs working in accent modification (Müller, Ball, & Guendouzi, 2000) despite the background and experience we bring to the table. In the end, both fields would be well-served to recognize their strengths and weakness and to acknowledge that anyone working in the world of accent modification needs to spend the time and devote the energy to mastering their craft. Most TESOL instructors will clearly need to acquire much of the technical knowledge that SLPs take for granted, but it is also important for professionals in our field to recognize some of the wonderful contributions to teaching sound systems (and especially suprasegmentals) that come from our TESOL colleagues. In fact, much of the research cited in this book, as well as many of the sources for ideas and materials, come from the TESOL world. In addition, many resources widely used by TESOL instructors throughout the world are not in common use by SLPs. *Well Said* (Grant, 2017) and *Targeting Pronunciation* (Miller, 2007), both written by SLPs for the TESOL market, are two examples. In some cases, SLPs work side by side with TESOL instructors or collaborate with them in programs, as I did when I worked at UCSD Exten-sion's English Language Institute. Figure 2–1 shows Paula Gallay, a licensed and certified SLP with over 25 years of experience, leading group work in a pronunciation class.

## Voice and Speech Trainers

Before discussing SLPs working in accent modification, there is one other category of professionals working in the field that encompasses individuals with all different types of backgrounds, who are not SLPs, but who provide individual or small group accent modification for a fee. These practitioners use a number of titles and descriptions, but perhaps the most common are dialect coach or accent trainer. They bring a wide range of experience and training, coming from all walks of life including the worlds of TESOL and drama training. These coaches work with clients on accent modification, and in some

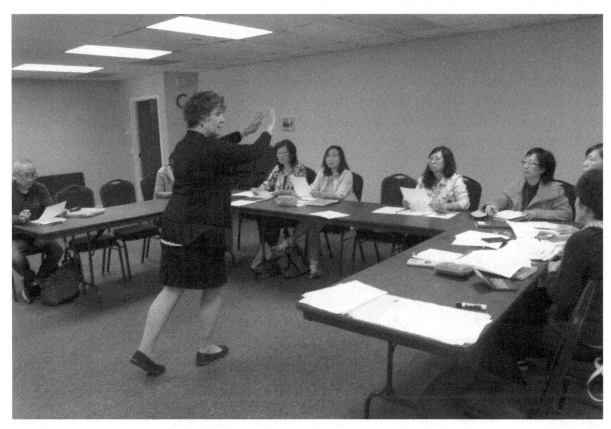

**Figure 2–1.** Paula Gallay leading a group.

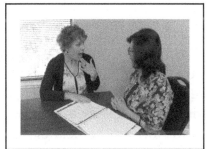

I worked in acute hospitals, rehabs, and transitional living centers. I've worked in private practice (pediatric and adult), public schools, and private schools.

About 7 years ago, I knew of an ESL program in my community that needed a teacher. It was an advanced ESL conversation class, and I was willing to try, but I informed the director that my skills were more suited to helping students pronounce English in a clear, understandable way. The director felt certain we did not need that in the program, that we just needed an ESL teacher. I invited her to come see my class and what I did to teach my students English pronunciation. After she saw what I do, and the results my students had, she understood I could offer a unique class that other ESL programs could not.

—Paula Gallay, M.S., CCC-SLP, AV Speech Therapy

cases, help actors create characters' voices based on dialects. They may also train non-native speakers in corporations in the United States or in other countries at call centers. The Voice and Speech Trainers Association (VASTA) is "a nonprofit, volunteer-driven organization dedicated to serving the needs of the voice and speech profession and to developing the art and science of the human voice," according to their website (https:// www.vasta.org/). Many of VASTA's members are engaged in accent modification, and while the majority of their members come from other fields, about 10% of their current 800 members are SLPs.

## Speech-Language Pathologists

SLPs and their colleagues in the world of TESOL share a love of language and a desire to improve communication, but several factors related to their scope of practice and training set their two professions apart. One major difference is that in contrast to TESOL teachers, SLPs do not generally provide accent modification services to children, who are still within the critical period for language acquisition and are expected to achieve nativelike proficiency without intervention. For example, a sixth-grade student from a culturally and linguistically diverse background who has average speech and language skills in their primary language but is still in the process of acquiring English phonology would be referred to the ELD department in a public school setting and would not receive speech and language services. However, it is entirely possible that in some cases, SLPs in a public school setting provide de facto accent modification for children who are on their caseloads due to delays in their primary language (or L1), and SLPs may also be called on to collaborate with ELD professionals, or even to provide some instruction within guidelines established by ASHA. Private SLP practitioners can provide accent modification to children or adolescents at their parents' request, but it is certainly not the norm in our field, while in the world of TESOL it is.

In terms of training, SLPs have much deeper knowledge of the anatomy and physiology of speech, and have a strong background in phonetics and transcription. ASHA requires that students entering graduate programs have taken an undergraduate phonetics class, and as a part of these courses, students learn a great deal of detail about the English sound system and how to transcribe it, including the intricacies of narrow transcription. In general, a strong background in phonetics is essential to work in the field of accent modification. Undergraduates also take classes that provide them with a background for studying speech disorders and aspects related to cultural and linguistic diversity, which can also help build a foundation for working on accent.

Students who are admitted to graduate programs may never again take a class as directly related to accent modification as phonetics, but much of their coursework will continue to shape their knowledge base for working with accents. Courses related to phonology, fluency, bilingualism, dysarthria, social language, as well as many others, will enable them to help non-native speakers communicate more effectively. In addition, graduate students receive extensive supervised clinical experience, which will hone their treatment skills. While it is typically uncommon for students to have a clinical placement

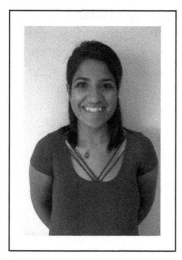

Phonetics was definitely the most helpful class because it taught me to listen to both segmental sounds and suprasegmental sounds. I love transcribing in IPA and it really helped that this was a skill that I had learned. My undergrad class required that we transcribe a language sample of someone whose second language was English. This also taught me to listen for differences in individuals' speech. I have always been interested in the differences between languages and the phonology of different languages, so accent was definitely an area of interest for me. I was excited to work with this unique population, especially because my parents and several extended family members have accents.

—Shefali Chauhan, Graduate Clinician

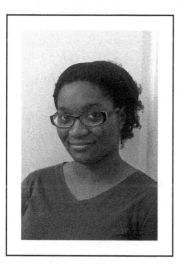

I believe that the language acquisition and phonetics/phonology classes that I took throughout college helped quite a bit. I understood the general idea of what it meant to have an accent as an adult, and I was able to apply what I learned about articulation and prosody in treating my clients. I think what helped me for one of my clients was being somewhat familiar with her primary language. During our sessions, I was able to not only recognize and understand how her primary language influenced her English, but I was also able to discuss those influences with her during session so that she could recognize them as well.

—Jessica Williams, Graduate Clinician

where they perform accent modification, it is highly likely that they will work on children's articulation, and this provides excellent training in shaping phoneme production. They may also work with clients on areas such as dysarthria, fluency, or prosody. When they are off campus at schools and hospitals, they will also work with clients and alongside fellow professionals who are non-native speakers. When viewed from any angle, the immersive training in all facets of communication and the many hours of clinical experience that graduate students receive in SLP programs gives them excellent preparation to provide effective accent modification services.

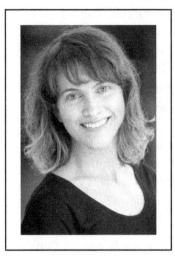

In graduate school, through the assessment of school-aged children, I learned about the phonology of other languages and what is shared between various languages and English. This knowledge carried over nicely into accent modification and knowing what types of errors a non-native English speaker could be expected to make. As a professional, working with speech and voice patients on respiration, phonation, resonance, and prosody/intonation helped the most.

—Julie Cunningham, M.A., CCC-SLP, San Diego Voice and Accent

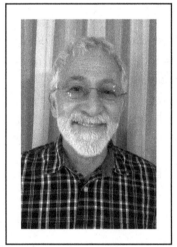

All of my graduate training helped in some way. Articulation/phonological disorders, fluency, and pragmatics have helped with all my clients. The one course outside of grad school that has helped the most is PROMPT (Prompts for Restructuring Oral Muscular Phonetic Targets). Giving direct physical prompts for th, t, g and r. Explaining vowel and jaw opening by using a 1-4 system seems to help clients produce correct vowels sounds easier.

—Steve Glance, M.S., CCC-SLP, Coast Speech Pathology

Despite this extensive preparation, it is common for SLPs entering the field to wonder if they need additional training or certification to provide accent modification services. Graduate programs are extremely rigorous, but because of the breadth of our field, they produce generalists with excellent knowledge and capabilities who will go on to develop highly specialized skills over time. As discussed above, because accents are not disorders, there is typically no requirement to have a license or degree to work with them, and there are no additional certifications required for SLPs to work on accent modification. At times,

As communication specialists, SLPs are uniquely qualified to provide accent modification training. SLPs take courses such as language development, articulation, phonetics, phonology, and the anatomy and physiology of speech & hearing mechanisms. We are trained in modifying, remediating and habilitating speech sound production. We've also received training in voice, and resonance, as well as the suprasegmental aspects of speech and language. These include word & sentence stress, intonation, rhythm, word linking, and word reductions. We know nonverbal communication also, such as volume, tone of voice, facial expression, and body language. We can take a holistic approach and train communication skills in order to refine and strengthen the whole package (verbal, nonverbal, and cultural skills). Our education includes years of training and fellowship work (working under another certified SLP) and continuing education hours every year. SLPs hold certification mandated by our state, and by the American Speech-Language-Hearing Association.

—Paula Gallay

SLPs will refer to being certified in accent training, but this always refers to a particular method promoted by an individual or company and not something that is required by ASHA. While many of these programs provide an excellent way for SLPs to hone their skills, and they may have additional marketing advantages for those who complete them, they are in no way a requirement to provide accent modification services. On the other hand, ASHA's Code of Ethics (ASHA, 2016) mandates that SLPs "shall engage in only those aspects of the professions that are within the scope of their professional practice and competence, considering their certification status, education, training, and experience," so it is essential that SLPs devote time and energy to bridge any gaps in their knowledge and develop the skills necessary to become first-class practitioners in the field of accent modification if they offer that service, and one of the aims of this book is to provide guidance to do just that.

## Where SLPs Practice Accent Modification

As mentioned above, a great deal of accent modification work is conducted in TESOL classrooms in the United States and throughout the world, but SLPs engaged in accent modification work primarily in private practice, at university clinics, or offer the service as a part of their other job duties. Those engaged in private practice may own or work in small clinics and see clients individually or in groups. Many practitioners have businesses on the internet where clients can access training materials or videos, and services are offered through telepractice. SLPs may operate as independent contractors and deliver services at companies both in their home country and abroad. Many large corporations in English-speaking countries have significant numbers of foreign-born employees and are often willing to invest in accent modification to improve communication, while companies or call centers in other countries that engage in continual communication with English speakers also hire accent trainers to improve performance. Some university clinics provide accent modification training as a part of their graduate programs. In this case, accent modification is conducted by graduate students under the supervision of a licensed SLP. Finally, some SLPs are tasked with providing services as a part of their regular job duties. An example of this might be a hospital-based SLP who trains non-native coworkers through either a formal or informal arrangement.

## Private Practice

According to ASHA's private practice survey from 2015, across private practitioners who treated adult patients, about 2% of their time was spent on accent modification. Some SLPs devote 100% of their time to providing accent modification services or training others to provide them, but many others engage in it as just a part of their private clinical practice or in addition to a full-time job. While many private clinics that work with children may hire SLPs immediately after they receive their degrees, accent modification practices tend to be smaller and are unlikely to be looking for fresh graduates to hire. Anecdotally, it is also rare for SLPs to begin working on accent modification until they are at least several years out of school. There are two typical pathways SLPs take toward full or part-time accent modification work in private practice. First, many SLPs enter the field after working in schools or hospitals because they are looking for something new and engaging. Second, many private practitioners begin accepting accent clients either to expand their practices, or because like their colleagues entering through the first pathway, they see it as a wonderful challenge.

SLPs working in private practice often see clients on a one-on-one basis in an office or clinic, but it is also common to provide services to small groups of three to five clients. In an article in *The ASHA Leader* entitled "A Growing Niche in Corporate America" (Feinstein-Whittaker, Wilner, & Sikorski, 2012), the authors advocate for consideration of the group approach, stating "successful trainers seeking a broad spectrum of corporate clients need to consider the financial and logistical needs of their clients and offer small (three to six participants) or midsize (seven to 12) groups." When working with larger groups, SLPs typically conduct the sessions at a company. In addition to practical advantages related to logistics and pricing, working with groups lets clinicians take advantage of a collaborative learning environment. In the group format, clinicians can often find a good price balance by decreasing the cost that each group member would pay individually, while still earning a higher hourly fee, and clients appreciate the lower price without a substantial decrease in attention from the clinician. While clinicians have provided accent modification by telepractice for many years, in the last decade this has become much more feasible due to improvements in technology. There are many platforms available that allow for transmission of high quality sound and video at a reasonable price, and telepractice is extremely practical considering the number of potential clients who live in other countries.

SLPs charge for their work, and rightly so, for they are highly qualified professionals providing services their clients' desire. Because accent is not a disability, these services are not covered by insurance, so individuals or the corporations they work for pick up the tab. There is really no going rate for accent modification services, since there are so many variables including geographic location, the SLP's experience and qualifications, the current market, and travel. As with any free market enterprise, the appropriate price is the one that client and clinician agree to.

## University Programs

Although some university clinics offer accent modification as an option for their students, they tend to be in the minority. When these services are offered, they are virtually always dwarfed by services for children and adults with disorders. It is also common for a particular supervisor to be assigned accent clients on an irregular basis. Accent programs are popular with graduate students training to be SLPs, especially those with some experience learning languages, and since these programs tend to be either free or low cost, they are popular with clients as well. In some cases, non-native-speaking graduate students in SLP programs receive accent modification at their own universities.

## Worksites

SLPs are often viewed as a resource when administrators are concerned about developing the English oral proficiency skills of their employees. Many years ago, I attended a weekend accent training workshop attended predominantly by SLPs, with a smattering of TESOL teachers and graduate students. During the introductions, one attendee explained that she was an SLP working in a hospital where many doctors, nurses, technicians, and other professionals were non-native speakers, and she had been tasked with developing a training program to help the staff communicate more effectively. I have heard many similar stories since, and it is clear that this occurs both formally and informally at many work settings that employ SLPs.

# How Does Accent Modification Work?

## Overview

Clinicians work with clients to make changes in their communication skills that can help them achieve their personal and professional goals. Training may focus on intelligibility, naturalness, fluency, pragmatics, voice and resonance, or any number of additional areas necessary to improve clients' communicative effectiveness. On the other hand, syntax and semantics are generally handled differently. Non-natives' usage of the target language will generally differ from that of natives in more than just accentedness, and this is often called interlanguage because it shares features of both languages. This interlanguage may feature semantic and syntactic differences that may have a profound effect on the communicative effectiveness of non-natives. Traditionally, SLPs have shied away from providing direct services to ameliorate these differences. ASHA's scope of practice (2016) discusses accent modification as addressing "sound pronunciation, stress, rhythm, and intonation of speech to enhance effective communication," and excludes crucial aspects of second language acquisition such as syntax and semantics. The implication is that nonphonological aspects should be left to our colleagues in the world of TESOL. There is certainly nothing wrong with helping clients in these nonphonology-related areas when problems arise during the course of services, but the focus is primarily on phonology. In some cases, pronunciation practice ties in with semantics or syntax, such as work on regular past tense endings or the use of idioms in teaching suprasegmentals. On a final note, there does not appear to be a true critical period for acquisition of native-like grammaticality judgment or vocabulary development. There are many examples of non-natives who equal or surpass their native-speaking peers in these aspects of English language proficiency.

In describing typical pronunciation work, Celce-Murcia and colleagues (2010) list the following as some of the typical training strategies:

- Listen and imitate
- Phonetic training
- Minimal pair drill (including contextualized minimal pairs)
- Visual aids (cues to assist in the production of sound)
- Tongue twisters
- Developmental approximation drills (following a developmental sequence in learning sounds of the L2)
- Vowel production practice and stress pattern alteration
- Reading aloud
- Recordings of client's production for auditory feedback and review

This list should in no way be considered exhaustive, and clinicians should use their imaginations and the ever-growing number of resources available to expand the range of strategies they use. Additional strategies include role-plays, dialogs, choral readings, shadowing, conversation starters, visual feedback, and auditory discrimination.

There is no set time frame for the length of training since clients have a wide variety of goals and abilities. In some cases, a client may be satisfied with one or two sessions, while others may continue training for many years. SLPs in private practice often provide training in packages with a set number of sessions, and in university programs, clients typically receive training for one or two semesters.

Much of the work that SLPs do can be divided into two levels: segmental and supra-segmental, and this book provides detailed analysis of assessment, target selection, and training ideas for both levels. SLPs come out of graduate school with an excellent understanding of segmentals, which represent the individual sounds of the language, especially in terms of the consonants. Much of the work done in accent modification involves vowels, in contrast to most of the work done by SLPs who work on articulation with children. Accent modification involves helping clients acquire or shape phonemes, which is familiar territory for SLPs with a strong background in articulation, but we also work a great deal on the allophones of English, which are much less important when working with native speakers. In terms of the suprasegmentals, SLPs may be less familiar, especially in terms of how they might analyze non-native variations from typical English patterns and then provide effective training to address them.

Syllables: Many English words are multisyllabic, and clients need to produce the words with the same number of syllables as natives typically do. For example, a speaker from Brazil might say the word *office* as [ɔfisi] with three syllables as opposed to two, which can affect intelligibility or naturalness. The number of syllables also ties into the regular past tense and *s* endings in English, so if a client from Argentina says *decided* as [disaɪd] native speakers might interpret it as referring to the present and not the past.

Stress: Multisyllabic English words have one syllable that stands out the most because it is stressed. If a Czech says *insurance* as ['ɪnʃɚɛnts] with stress on the first syllable and not the second, it may lead to a misunderstanding. In addition, a client from Japan might say the word *biology* with much less variation in pitch and it will sound unnatural.

Linking: In English, we connect the sounds within a phrase, so a client from China might say *in about an hour* with glottal stops between each word, whereas native speakers connect these words without a break. In addition, when we link our sounds, some allophonic rules come into play, so the /t/ in *about* becomes an alveolar tap when we connect it to a word beginning with a vowel.

Phrasal stress: English speakers use a rhythm that might be different from that of our clients' native language (L1). One important feature is that we suppress the stress on many words within a sentence, especially the function words, such as articles and prepositions. If a client from Thailand puts stress on every word in the sentence *I went to the store*, it will sound choppy. English speakers would normally put tonic stress on *store* and a touch of stress on *went*, but the other words would be destressed.

Emphasis: Every language has different ways of calling attention to particular elements of an utterance, and in English this is usually done with stress. If we think of the previous sentence *I went to the store*, we mentioned that stress would normally go on *store*, but if someone asks the question, "Who went to the store?" then stress would normally shift to *I* in the answer. In theory, stress can be shifted to any element of a phrase, so a speaker might say "I went TO the store" and jump up on the preposition to indicate that he didn't come *from* the store. While this may seem obvious to native speakers of English, our clients speak languages that achieve this effect through different means and they may need to develop awareness of our model.

Reduced vowels: Another feature of English is that vowels are often reduced when they are destressed. A client from Korea might use the /æ/ vowel in the word *can* in the sentence *I can go now*, while a native speaker would reduce it to a schwa or elide it entirely and use a syllabic /n/.

Rate: There is a general conception that native speakers should slow down in order to be better understood, but the evidence does not bear this out, and the impact of reduced rate on naturalness can outweigh any possible gains. Native speakers almost always speak faster than non-native speakers, and our clients virtually always speak more slowly in English than they do when speaking their own language. The goal should be a natural sounding rate that best promotes intelligibility, but in general this should involve speaking faster.

Intonation: This book uses the term *intonation* in a narrower sense than *prosody* to refer to the melody of speech. This can be one of the most important factors in helping clients sound more natural. Each language has its own patterns of intonation, and there is an incredible amount of variation across languages. The way we say something is often just as important as what we are saying, and intonation plays an oversized role in conveying the true meaning of our words.

Voice and resonance do not fit squarely into the segmental or suprasegmental categories, but they often have an important role in accent modification and SLPs need no prompting to address them. Some clients may have voice issues that are unrelated to their accent, but you may also notice aspects of voice or resonance that differ due to L1 interference. For example, clients who speak languages that use nasality phonemically or have a large number of nasalized vowels, such as Polish, French, or Portuguese, may sound hypernasal in English. This book does not address this topic in detail because there are so many books available on the topic of voice and all the training SLPs have regarding voice applies more or less directly to their work in accent modification. SLPs are trained to play close attention to differences in voice and nasality, and they have the background, training, and resources to address them as part of their work. The last aspect to address is what we call *pragmatics*, which in this case can be better labeled *communication style*. As a part of accent training, clinicians usually consider not just the specific speaking style of each client, but also how cultural norms relating to gestures and body language influence communication in English.

## Counseling

ASHA's website lists "counseling persons seeking accent modification services regarding communication-related issues" as an appropriate role for SLPs, yet this topic is almost never addressed in the accent modification literature. Perhaps this is because a great deal of the work related to accent training comes from the world of TESOL, where this is not a consideration. The connection may not always be readily apparent. One of the graduate students I was supervising in our Accent and Communication Training program at SDSU approached me at the beginning of the year because she had been assigned a project to write about her counseling experiences when working with clients during the semester, and she wanted to know if counseling would play enough of a role in her sessions to provide material for her assignment. I told her it would, and at the conclusion of the program she told me how surprised she was at the amount of counseling she actually did. Some of the counseling may be relatively light, such as suggestions for practice opportunities or discussions of strategies, but at other times, the counseling can be deep and relate to issues of clients' self-esteem, feelings of inadequacy, or isolation.

In order to counsel our clients, we have to feel compassion for them, so it is important to revisit some of the issues addressed at the very beginning of this book, related to accent and identity. We all take for granted the feeling of group identity that speaking in our native accent gives us. My first real personal experiences with accent came when I studied abroad in West Germany as a UCLA undergraduate in the early 1980s. I had always assumed that with enough practice I would sound like a native, and yet the second I spoke in German people knew I was not one. Just as many people who stutter do, I would sometimes keep quiet when I entered a store because I wanted to fit in and I felt I would be labeled by those who heard me speak. Gradually, I came to accept that it was better to communicate openly and try not to worry about what others might notice. Many of the feelings that people who stutter have are shared by those who speak with an accent every day, and SLPs who have experience working with these clients can apply some of the insights they have gained from that work. Non-natives often feel that they are never able to join the club, and these feelings can lead to a sense of isolation.

Non-natives understand the incredible challenges involved in mastering another language, and yet many native speakers who have never taken the time to learn another language will judge them to be less intelligent based on their accent or second language proficiency. Feeling judged as inferior is a staggeringly common perception among native speakers despite its fundamental illogic, and these perceptions can be especially challenging for non-natives who have mastered the grammar, vocabulary, and even the phonology of a language, but may still have high accentedness ratings. In the words of one of my clients when asked how she feels in this kind of situation, "It is not your first language. Many people only speak one language, and you are trying another one so of course, it's hard. I hope Americans don't see the accent as a sign of stupidity because we can only try our best! Do they speak another language as well as I speak English?"

Clients also report differences in the attitudes of interlocutors based on the client's native language. For example, clients whose L1 is French may be told how wonderful their accent is, while a speaker of Chinese might only hear negative comments, even if their relative accentedness is the same. These biases are largely the result of native speakers' perceptions of the client's country or culture, and they represent an additional level of bias that must be overcome. Even for speakers with "prestige" non-native accents, the positive comments may be patronizing and can involve inaccurate preconceptions.

Language is so central to our identity that we feel our words are who we are. Many non-natives report that when they speak in their L2, they feel like they are wearing a mask, and that it is impossible to reveal their true identity. This can lead to frustration and the feeling that colleagues and even loved ones may never know who they really are. Wearing the mask takes effort as well; non-natives need to put in extra effort when they speak their L2 and must pay more attention to whether others are following along with what they are saying. They also have to be on the lookout for any potentially embarrassing mistakes that can lead to mockery or derision. The balance of power can shift quickly when native speakers point out that a word was pronounced incorrectly. Clients have reported situations in which they have given lengthy presentations they felt were successful, and then when someone commented on the way they pronounced a particular word or phrase, the client suddenly felt inadequate.

Non-native speakers have a host of reasons for moving to another country and needing to speak a second language. Many have strong intrinsic motivation to assimilate to the greatest extent possible, but others may not feel the same urge. Someone who had always been excited about learning English and living in this country is likely to have substantially different motivation to have a sense of belonging than someone who is here because a spouse was sent on assignment for a two-year stint. In addition, the desire to be accepted in the new language might bring feelings of a loss of culture or even betrayal of a native culture. Sometimes clients report that they do not want to lose their identity by changing their accent. An outsider might view this as a type of defensive reaction, but that really misses the point. Non-natives often feel a sense of conflicting pressure to choose between identities related to their L1 as opposed to their L2. We can say that they do not have to make a choice, but to some extent they do. Gatbonton, Trofimovich, and Magid (2005) reported that L1-speaking peers sometimes considered speakers who strove to adopt a more native sounding accent in their L2 were being disloyal to their compatriots. We can counsel clients about the advantages of modifying their accents, but we have to recognize the complexities involved.

Apart from these more abstract personal feelings and perceptions of others, there is concrete evidence illustrating the many forms of discrimination non-native speakers face. Baugh (2003) used the same actors to speak in Standard American English and to imitate native speakers of different languages and dialects in order to compare responses to inquiries about housing. There was a correlation between the dialect used by the actor and the reported availability of housing, indicating that there was a bias against accents which strayed from the prestige dialect. Lev-Ari and Keysar (2010) demonstrated that statements read by non-natives were deemed less credible than those read by natives, even when judges were explicitly told that the statements did not originate with the speakers. Remarkably, Hanzlíková and Sarnitzl (2017) found this same effect for non-native judges.

---

It's important to remember that when teaching accent modification, SLPs are never trying to eliminate someone's self, personality or cultural identity. And accent is never bad. Accent tells a listener that a person grew up in a specific place, or among a specific cultural community. It is only when an accent gets in the way of communication that we work to help clients use the expected sounds and patterns of English. The Standard American English accent can be learned whether someone grew up speaking Mandarin Chinese or with a regional dialect like a Boston accent or a southern U.S. accent. SLPs should never strive to take away a client's identity. We only help them learn to *code switch* easily between Standard American English and their first language or dialect.

—Paula Gallay

Anecdotally, many clients report a belief that their accent interfered with their ability to get a job, and unfortunately, there is evidence bearing this out. Munro (2003) found instances of employment and housing discrimination, as well as harassment, based on accent in a review of human rights cases in Canada. Carlson and McHenry (2006) showed that a person's ethnicity did not affect employment prospects unless they spoke with a significant accent. Most non-natives do, of course, get jobs, but it is difficult to gauge how their accents affected the choices available to them. In addition, clients often report fears that they will not receive promotions as readily as their native-speaking colleagues. Fuertes and colleagues (2012, p. 130) wrote, "In closing, evaluations based on accent appear to have a significant impact on individuals who do not speak with standard accents and are likely to lead to discrimination and possibly other severe social consequences." In the same paper, Fuertes et al. reported that the perception of additional obstacles can create a self-fulfilling prophesy in terms of poor performance when non-natives are concerned about possible bias on the part of listeners.

Many clients seek accent modification because they have jobs that require a great deal of speaking. In some professions, such as those in the tech field, a large number of professionals are non-native speakers and collaboration occurs through emails and reports, although oral proficiency can still be a determining factor in advancement. In the teaching profession, on the other hand, the oral component is almost always pivotal. Faculty and graduate assistants frequently report that students give them low evaluations based on their accents, and it is reasonable to assume that bias plays a role.

Our profession itself is not above reproach in terms of accent bias and discrimination. Several case studies were reported in an ASHA Professional Issues Statement from 2011 involving graduate students who overcame barriers on their paths to becoming SLPs because of their accents. Some were discouraged from continuing in the major or told that their only career path option was research. All are now highly respected practitioners. ASHA's position is that non-native-speaking students and professionals can provide services as long as they have "the expected level of knowledge in normal and disordered communication, the expected level of diagnostic and clinical case management skills, and if modeling is necessary, the ability to model the target phoneme, grammatical feature, or other aspect of speech and language that characterizes the client's particular problem" (ASHA, 1991). The need for our profession to attract and train non-native speakers to be

---

The clients I usually see are struggling to keep their jobs or are interviewing for a new position. They are not understood at work and are having significant work-related problems. We focus on vocabulary from their work or a typical work report. Right now I work with civil engineers so I pull interview questions and articles from Google about civil engineering projects. It's terrific to work with someone and see the improvement.

—Steve Glance

clinicians is particularly important given the changing demographics of our country and a lack of bilingual SLPs. We owe it to our clients to go out of our way to support these students and help them join our ranks.

In addition to those outlined above, the list of potential impacts non-native speakers face because of their accents is truly limitless, and there are many that they may be either unaware of or hesitant to discuss. Clients will often discuss day-to-day problems such as difficulties ordering the exact type of coffee they want, but they may not feel comfortable bringing up the effect their accent might have on their ability to enter into a relationship or make friends.

SLPs should keep these considerations in the back of their minds when working with non-native speakers. Most clients do not come to accent modification with the intention of having lengthy counseling sessions about the challenges they face in their personal or professional lives, but these factors are always lingering beneath the surface and SLPs should be ready to listen and lend support. Listening is truly the most impor-

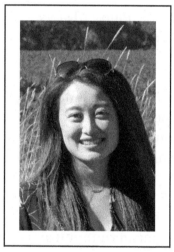

As a non-native speaker of English, I am more sensitive to how the phonology and syntax of the first language impacts the acquisition of a second language (e.g., phoneme substitutions, cluster reduction, pro-drop). It gives me specific areas to target when providing my therapy. Our field is in need of more bilingual SLPs and I would tell any non-native speakers entering our profession not to be afraid of having an accent. Being a non-native speaker means you need to make an extra effort, but don't be afraid. Work harder and make yourself shine. You are the unicorn many school districts, hospitals, and private practices are looking for.

—Alice Li, Graduate Clinician

Though I really appreciate all the support and help I've gotten from instructors, cohorts, and other clinicians, as a non-native speaker who studies English as a second language and dreams to become an SLP, it is way harder to succeed in the clinical field than a local student can imagine. The language barrier is obviously a big challenge and no one else except myself can help with that. I hope in the future, there will be more ways for non-native speakers to pursue their SLP dreams with less trouble.

—Yiyang Shen, Graduate Clinician

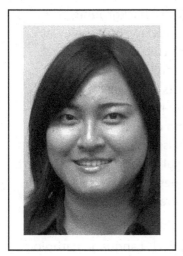

As a non-native speaker in my undergraduate and graduate Communication Sciences and Disorders (CSD) programs, the biggest challenge I faced was overcoming my fear of sounding different and learning how to be comfortable with my accent. I constantly worried that by speaking with an accent that deviates from Standard American English and making occasional grammatical errors, I would present myself as a less intelligent person. As a result, I feared public speaking. This fear contributed to my lack of courage to participate more in classes throughout my undergraduate and graduate studies. As a non-native-speaking clinician/student in the CSD field, always come more prepared than you think you were. One important tip I would like to share is to be confident. As a non-native speaker, you definitely have a lot to share and teach about your native language, so don't be afraid to speak up in class and let your voice be heard. Instead of being concerned about your accent, be proud of yourself as a future bilingual speech-language pathologist!

—Wen-Hsin Ku, Graduate Clinician

tant part of the counseling process. SLPs can represent a crucial bridge between the worlds of native and non-native speakers, acting as a type of accent confidante. Clients often report how much they enjoy discussing the technical aspects of L2 phonology with someone who understands it and can explain it to them. When native speakers point out a pronunciation error, they are usually at a loss to explain how to overcome it, apart from providing a quick model. SLPs also have good backgrounds in counseling and in the social and emotional impacts of communication difficulties, and they can use their experience to help clients overcome a variety of challenges. There is no need to sugarcoat the problems non-native speakers face because of their accents. By listening compassionately, SLPs can help clients move forward with a realistic but positive attitude and focus on the aspects of their communication their clients have the power to change.

## Terminology

Accent modification currently appears to be the most acceptable description for services designed to change adult speakers' second language phonology and this is the term used by ASHA. There have been many terms used synonymously over the years, such as *accent*

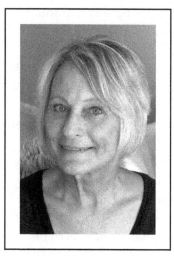

Working with clients from very diverse backgrounds requires cultural sensitivity and a global worldview. Because I was exposed to and embraced different cultures from a very young age, my comfort level with multiple languages, social mores, values, and customs of clients is a given. It's been relatively easy to establish trust and rapport and to put clients at ease. Some clients have no one else to talk with about communication and cultural issues they encounter at work, within their family, or in social situations. As an accent reduction professional, one often becomes the go-to person for clients who are trying to navigate a culture that may be new to them.

—Pat Chien, Speech-Language Pathologist,
American Accent Specialties

---

It's important to remember that when teaching accent modification, SLPs are never trying to eliminate someone's self, personality, or cultural identity. And accent is never bad. Accent tells a listener you grew up in a specific place, or within a specific cultural community. It is only when your accent gets in the way of communication that we work to help you use the expected sounds and patterns of English. The Standard American English accent can be learned whether you grew up speaking Mandarin Chinese, or with a regional dialect like a Boston accent or a southern U.S. accent. We never strive to take away your identity. We only help you learn to code switch easily between Standard American English and your first language/dialect.

—Paula Gallay

---

*reduction, accent coaching, accent enhancement,* and *accent addition.* The term *accent reduction* has fallen out of favor because of its implication that the non-native accent should be reduced or eliminated. *Modification* is a more neutral term which simply implies making changes to increase communicative effectiveness. Opinions vary on these terms, and SLPs may also need to evaluate marketing aspects or other considerations when selecting a description of their services. Many who work with accent modification try to avoid using descriptors such as *good, bad, thick,* and *beautiful* when referring to accents because they seek a more neutral approach that views accent only in terms of its impact on communication. Nevertheless, it is extremely common to hear these adjectives applied even by the clients themselves. In addition, because accents represent natural differences and not disorders, much of the terminology normally used in the field of speech-language pathology is not applicable. Terms such as *disorder, delay,* and *disability* do not apply since we expect adults to have an accent when they learn a second language, and there are no norms about how adults should progress as they acquire a second phonology. Replacing the word *therapy* is important but difficult, and one of the more popular terms in use is *training*.

The terms used in the TESOL community are somewhat different. While the term *accent* is in common use, *accent modification* is almost never used, and instead, *pronunciation* and *pronunciation instruction* are vastly more common. Logically, *student* is the term of choice rather than *client*. Most of the terms used to describe phonological features are shared, with a few exceptions based on preference. For example, in the TESOL world *fluency* is used much more commonly than in speech-language pathology with regard to second language learning, since TESOL professionals do not associate that word with stuttering as SLPs do, and *prosody* is almost never used by teachers.

## Who Are Our Clients?

Clients seek accent modification for a variety of reasons, but in general they are highly motivated and seek services because they view their accent as an impediment to success. SLPs generally work with adult clients who voluntarily seek services or have been enrolled in a program by an employer. In the school system, SLPs do not typically work with non-native-speaking children because accents represent a difference not a disorder, and they would not be eligible to receive services. A typically developing non-native-speaking child who faces difficulties communicating at school because of an accent would be served by an English language development department. In such cases, SLPs often find themselves educating other professionals as to SLP roles and responsibilities. A student who communicates effectively in a language other than English is not an appropriate candidate for special education services in the area of speech and language and should not receive accent modification as a part of an Individualized Education Plan.

In addition to the commonality of being non-disordered non-native-speaking adults, clients tend to share several other characteristics. They tend to be highly motivated, although it is also possible that they are being asked to take part in a program at the request of their employer. Most clients are students or professionals, although spouses of professionals who have moved to the country frequently seek services as well. Many teachers, professors, and graduate assistants become clients, because of the importance of oral communication in their work, but I have worked with doctors, lawyers, homemakers, artists, filmmakers, engineers, and Uber drivers, to name a few additional occupations. It is possible to list the major L1 languages spoken by clients as a general tendency, and Table 2–1 is an attempt to do so, but the numbers depend on many variables, such as location, current economic conditions, and type of accent practice involved. Clients can truly come from any country or speak any language, but this represents a snapshot of the most common ones overall, with a ballpark estimate of frequency indicated by the order.

Languages, and not countries, are listed in Table 2–1 since that is most relevant for our work, but there will obviously be major differences in frequency of the various

**Table 2–1.** Common Client Languages for Accent Modification

| 1 | Chinese (both Mandarin and Cantonese) |
|---|---|
| 2 | Spanish |
| 3 | Korean |
| 4 | Russian |
| 5 | Japanese |
| 6 | Indian languages (both Indo-European and Dravidian) |
| 8 | Arabic |
| 9 | Persian |
| 10 | Vietnamese |
| 11 | French |
| 12 | Turkish |
| 13 | Thai |
| 14 | German |
| 15 | Portuguese |
| 16 | Polish |

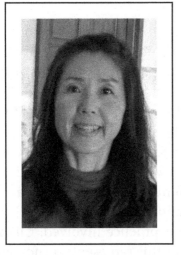

I chose accent modification because I get self-conscious and nervous talking to native speakers largely because of pronunciation and grammatical mistakes I might make. I wanted to feel more competent and confident about my pronunciation. The sessions helped me to raise my overall awareness of what to watch for. For example, I became aware how I had been omitting pronouncing mid and final r's, or how important it was to reduce insignificant syllables. I understand that it takes effort to communicate with someone who has an accent, and I don't blame native speakers who lose interest or feel slightly annoyed by communicating with people with an accent. I'd like them to focus on the points we are trying to convey, even when those points are being delivered in rough, less than perfect packaging.

—Saeko Inoue, Accent Modification Client

nationalities that speak a particular language. Despite the significant differences between Mandarin and Cantonese, and the Indo-European and Dravidian languages of India, they are lumped together because they are in the same *sprachbund* and share many features significant for accent work.

Clients who elect accent training understand that they will need to invest time and money and are therefore likely to feel a sense of urgency. They may feel some stress related to their accent and its effect on their personal or professional lives; many clients will share these feelings openly. This is not to suggest that accent clients are morose. While many SLPs enjoy some of the linguistic and phonological aspects of accent modification, the clients are truly the biggest draw to this subfield, and sometimes lifelong connections are formed.

# Does Accent Modification Work?

## Efficacy Studies

When I was in graduate school examining the evidence related to the acquisition of L2 phonology, the literature frequently referred to the dearth of research, but in the last few decades the landscape has changed. There is more and more evidence that positive outcomes can be achieved through accent training. Investigations of the efficacy of accent modification have gone through several stages, and there has recently been a sharp jump in the number of studies examining the effectiveness of pronunciation instruction. Most of the work sited below focuses on second language learning, and while most involve pronunciation teachers, and not SLPs providing accent modification services, the applicability is generally clear.

At the time of writing, two important metastudies stand out, and both demonstrated positive effects. Saito reviewed 15 quasi-experimental intervention studies published since 1990,  and found that "all intervention studies demonstrated significant improvement resulting from instruction except two studies" (Saito, 2012, p. 846). The two studies that failed to show gains involved mechanical drills without practice in broader, less structured activities. The studies showed efficacy in terms of both listener judgments of comprehensibility and specific aspects of L2 phonology at both the segmental and suprasegmental levels. On a side note, one of the studies reviewed, conducted by Saito and Lyster (2012), showed strong gains for Japanese learners working to acquire /ɹ/, and this may be of particular interest for SLPs working with Japanese speaking clients. Lee, Jang, and Plonsky (2015) reviewed 86 studies and found a large effect for pronunciation instruction, stating that "the learners who received instructional treatments improved by 0.89 standard deviation units in comparison with their pretreatment performance; the between-group analyses demonstrated that learners in experimental groups outperformed those in control groups by 0.80 standard deviation units," which according to the authors, represents medium to large effects (Lee, Jang, & Plonsky, 2015, pp. 356–357).

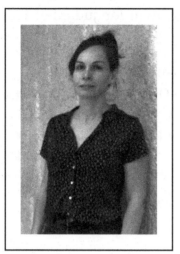

I had just moved to the US and I was looking for a job, and I thought if I could improve my accent I would have a better chance of getting a job. Accent modification helped me realize that one's accent doesn't need to disappear in order to be understood; if you have an accent and have clear pronunciation you will be understood. And I believe that if you are dedicated and try hard you can definitely improve your pronunciation and become clearer to be understood by everyone.

—Aurelia Viard, Accent Modification Client

As a working professional with customer meetings daily across the USA, I received feedback from my management that my accent was becoming an issue and needed to be addressed. The problem was mostly present for accounts located in states that are less exposed to foreigners. As a result, I was asked to provide a solution and work on correcting my pronunciation if I wanted to maintain all my accounts. After 2 months of sessions, I started receiving feedback from customers on the clarity of my explanations during conference calls, and I could feel more confident picking up the phone and calling a customer instead of sending an email. I've witnessed progress already and I received all the tools I need to keep making progress for tomorrow.

—Neila Guetat, Accent Modification Client

At this juncture, there is another aspect of research to address: the relative efficacy of pronunciation instruction aimed at the segmental versus the suprasegmental level. Over the years, this has been a subject of debate within the TESOL research community, but much of the discussion appears to have come as a result of a misinterpretation of one of the most important early studies in the literature (Derwing, Munro, & Wiebe, 1998; Derwing & Rossiter, 2003). The study analyzed the efficacy of pronunciation instruction by comparing a control group to one that focused on suprasegmentals and to another on segmentals, for accuracy, fluency, and complexity. The results showed gains for both types of pronunciation instruction and demonstrated better generalization in the supra-segmental group. Since that point, many researchers have weighed in on the segmentals versus suprasegmentals debate even though the authors of the original study have stated that they had only hoped to investigate the effects in isolation and were never advocating for an artificial dichotomy (Derwing & Munro, 2015). Since Saito (2012) as well as Lee, Jang, and Plonsky (2015) showed positive outcomes for work at both levels in their meta-analyses, SLPs should always consider both levels to address their clients' individual needs, and that philosophy is a central tenet of this book.

A study conducted by Khurana and Huang (2013), which was not included in either of the metastudies, may have some added applicability to SLPs working in accent modification. Although this study did not examine SLPs providing accent modification services, the providers were private-sector practitioners with TESOL backgrounds, who specialized in accent modification. Moreover, the program was provided on-site to medical professionals, which more closely reflects the work of SLPs in the field. A statistical analysis of the subjects' pre- and posttraining self-evaluations showed higher ratings after accent modification, with the greatest impact coming in terms of increased confidence. This last point is particularly important for our services because clients determine whether accent modification works by choosing it and reporting positive outcomes. While objective measurements of increased intelligibility or naturalness are important, clients' improved confidence in their own communication skills is another sign of success.

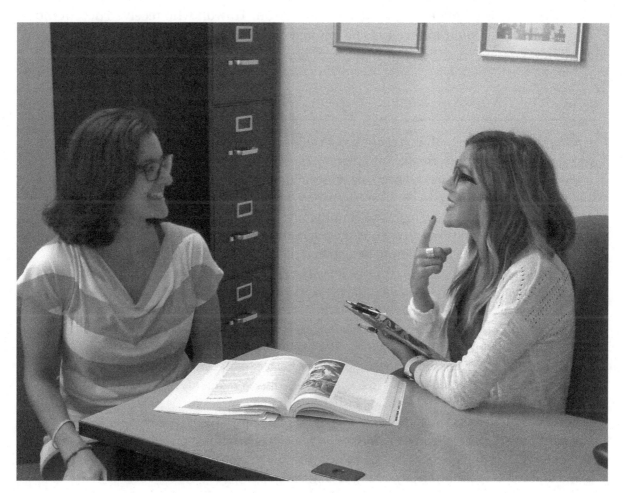

**Figure 2–2.** Neila Guetat with her graduate clinician Alexa Cavalea.

## Non-Native Clinicians

Those who speak English with a non-native accent may wonder if they can provide effective accent modification services, and the answer is a resounding yes! Having a non-native accent does not in and of itself prevent anyone from providing outstanding services in any area of practice, including accent modification. Evidence to support this comes from the world of TESOL, since it is very common in that field for non-natives to work on accent. Levis, Sonsaat, Link, and Barriuso (2016) conducted a study comparing pronunciation classes provided by native and non-native speakers and found similar results for both teacher types in terms of changes in the students' accentedness and intelligibility.

However, in contrast to the vast number of non-native TESOL teachers who provide quality pronunciation work to their students throughout the world, relatively few non-native SLPs even consider it an option, and there are several reasons for this, probably the most important of which relates to client expectations. In Levis et al. (2016), results were achieved in spite of the fact that many of the students had a stated preference for teachers who were native speakers. Thus, non-native speakers may face client bias in favor of native speakers when providing accent modification in languages other than their mother tongue.

Wen-Hsin Ku is a native speaker of Mandarin from Taiwan who received accent modification as an undergraduate before she entered a graduate SLP program, at which point she provided accent modification services to non-native clients as part of her supervised

---

Having the experience both as a client and a clinician in the accent program gave me a strong sense of empowerment. Transitioning to the role of a clinician from the role of a client empowered me and boosted my self-confidence as a non-native speaker. Since a clinician must be able to provide clear instructions and model segmental and suprasegmental targets, serving as a clinician in the accent program reassured me of my ability to juggle between managing my own accent and modeling the Standard American English accent. Having experience as a client before serving as a clinician in the accent program provided many other advantages as well. First of all, I was able to plan and execute the sessions based on what worked well and what didn't work as well in my own accent modification experience as a client. Second, as a fellow non-native speaker just like my clients, there was a tremendous buy-in for me as a clinician, especially when we shared the same native language. Sharing my firsthand experience as a client in the accent program with my clients allowed me to relate to the struggles they have experienced with their accent and gave me an understanding of how to counsel them during moments of frustration. It was also relatively easier for me to provide instructions and examples for Mandarin-speaking clients because of my understanding of Mandarin phonology as a native speaker. One of the most helpful things I learned as a client in the accent modification program and as a student in CSD is that everyone has an accent. The key to being a successful and effective communicator is speaking clearly and naturally, with or without a foreign accent.

—Wen-Hsin Ku

clinical experience. She is currently practicing as a school-based SLP, and she shares her perspective as someone who has sat on both sides of the table.

## A Note on Dialects

Students of linguistics quickly discover that the word *dialect* is notoriously difficult to define. Operationally, it tends to be defined as mutually intelligible versions of a language that can vary in terms of phonology, syntax, and semantics, among other factors. In reality, we know that someone speaking Swedish can converse with someone speaking Norwegian, even though both are defined as languages, while a fluent conversation between speakers of certain Chinese dialects would be very difficult. The dialects of English are also defined arbitrarily, and they can be broken down into any number of meaningful groupings, all of which are essentially abstractions. We have major distinctions, such as American English, British English, Australian English, and Indian English, and these can then be broken down into hundreds of regional and social dialects. When working with accent, it is common for clients to choose a prestige dialect as a model for their own pronunciation because these versions, by definition, are thought to provide a greater chance of success in society. In the United States, the version that is considered to be most widely used and least likely to face bias is sometimes called Standard American English, shortened to SAE, or sometimes General American English, abbreviated as GAE. Unfortunately, as Rosina Lippi-Green points out in her book *English with an Accent* (2012, p. 57), the notion of a standard form is an artificial construct. In her words, "nonlinguists are quite comfortable with the idea of a standard language, so much so that the average person is very willing to describe and define it, much in the same way that most people could draw a unicorn." In other words, we can all agree on what it is in theory, but that does not make it real. She herself has experimented with several terms to describe this "unicorn," including Standard American English and Mainstream English, and has now settled on *SAE with the asterisk denoting its fundamental inauthenticity.

This book focuses predominantly on the variety of English the above terms are meant to describe, which is the version most commonly heard on national news broadcasts in the United States, and is characterized by features such as rhoticity and the alveolar tap. We refer to this version as *American English*, especially when discussing features that are distinct from other major varieties of English such as British English, with the full understanding that the term *American English* is often used as an umbrella term that includes all of the dialects spoken in the U.S. There is no intention to promote this mythical version of English as superior to any other dialect, but instead, it is used as a placeholder for the typical dialect clients and clinicians often choose as a model in the U.S. Clinicians may need to adapt some of the materials (especially with regards to vowels) to match the version of English they speak or the version their clients would like to focus on. Clinicians from other English-speaking countries should also benefit from most of the information in this book, but will need to adapt more carefully.

SLPs also frequently provide dialect modification services to native speakers of English who speak a regional or social dialect and wish to modify their speech to sound more like another dialect of American English. Much of the information in this book applies to this type of work as well, but the primary focus remains on non-native speakers, rather than dialect speakers, and there are some key differences between the two. First, dialect speakers are able to function in English within specific contexts (whether geographic or social) with no communicative disadvantage, and second, there does not appear to be a critical period for native English speakers to acquire other English dialects. Many native speakers are able to acquire other dialects of English as adults at a level unmatched by their non-native peers. There is one final consideration concerning dialect clients. Any individual who seeks services voluntarily should be welcomed with open arms, but in some cases, a native speaker may be referred for training because of a regional or social dialect, and the clinician has an ethical obligation to investigate this situation with the client to determine if the referral is appropriate, since there is a strong potential that discrimination is involved.

# References

American Speech-Language-Hearing Association (1991). *Students and professionals who speak English with accents and nonstandard dialects: Issues and recommendations* [Position statement]. Retrieved from http://www.asha.org/policy/PS1998-00117/

American Speech-Language-Hearing Association (2011). *The clinical education of students with accents* [Professional issues statement]. Retrieved from http://www.asha.org/policy/PI2011-00324/

American Speech-Language-Hearing Association (2016). *Code of ethics.* Retrieved from http://www.asha.org/policy/

American Speech-Language-Hearing Association (2016). Scope of practice in speech-language pathology. Retrieved from http://www.asha.org/policy/

Baugh, J. (2003). Linguistic profiling. In S. Makoni, G. Smitherman, A. F. Ball, & A. K. Spears (Eds.) *Black linguistics: Language, society, and politics in Africa and the Americas,* (pp. 155–168). New York, NY: Routledge.

Carlson, H., & McHenry, M. (2006). Effect of accent and dialect on employability. *Journal of Employment Counselling, 43*(2), 70–83.

Celce-Murcia, M., Brinton, D., & Goodwin, J. M. (2010). *Teaching pronunciation: A course book and reference guide.* New York, NY: Cambridge University Press.

Derwing, T., & Munro, M. (2015). *Pronunciation fundamentals: Evidence-based perspectives for L2 teaching and research.* Philadelphia, PA: John Benjamins Publishing Company.

Derwing, T. M., Munro, M. J., & Wiebe, G. (1998). Evidence in favor of a broad framework for pronunciation instruction. *Language Learning, 48*(3), 393–410.

Derwing, T. M., & Rossiter, M. J. (2003). The effects of pronunciation instruction on the accuracy, fluency, and complexity of L2 accented speech. *Applied Language Learning, 13*(1), 1–18.

Feinstein-Whittaker, M., Wilner, L. K., & Sikorski, L. D. (2012). A growing niche in corporate America. *The ASHA Leader, 17,* 28–31.

Fuertes, J. N., Gottdiener, D. H., Martin, H., Gilbert, T. C., & Giles, H. (2012). A meta-analysis of the effects of speakers' accents on interpersonal evaluations. *European Journal of Social Psychology 42,* 120–133.

Gatbonton, E., Trofimovich, P., & Magid, M. (2005). Learners' ethnic group affiliation and L2 pronunciation accuracy: A sociolinguistic investigation. *TESOL Quarterly, 39*(3), 489–512.

Hanzlíková, D., & Skarnitzl, R. (2017). Credibility of native and non-native speakers of English revisited: Do non-native listeners feel the same? *Research in Language, 15,* 285–298. 10.1515/rela-2017-0016.

Khurana, P., & Huang, E. (2013). Efficacy of accent modification training for international medical professionals. *Journal of University Teaching & Learning Practice, 10*(2), 1–11.

Lee, J., Jang J., & Plonsky, L. (2015). The effectiveness of second language pronunciation instruction: A meta-analysis. *Applied Linguistics, 36*(3), 345–366.

Lev-Ari, S., & Keysar, B. (2010). Why don't we believe non-native speakers? The influence of accent on credibility. *Journal of Experimental Social Psychology, 46*(6), 1093–1096.

Levis, J. M., Sonsaat, S., Link, S., & Barriuso, T. A. (2016). Native and nonnative teachers of L2 pronunciation: Effects on learner performance. *TESOL Quarterly, 50*(4), 1–38.

Levy, E. S., & Crowley, C. J. (2011). Policies and practices regarding students with accents in speech-language pathology training programs. *Communication Disorders Quarterly, 34*(1), 59–68.

Lippi-Green, R. (2012). *English with an accent: Language, ideology and discrimination in the United States.* London, UK: Routledge.

Müller, N., Ball, M., & Guendouzi, J. (2000). Accent reduction programmes: Not a role for speech-language pathologists? *Advances in Speech Language Pathology, 2*(2) 119–129.

Munro, M. J. (2003). A primer on accent discrimination in the Canadian context. *TESL Canada Journal, 20*(2), 38–51.

Murphy, J. (2014). Teacher training programs provide adequate preparation in how to teach pronunciation. In Grant, L.J., *Pronunciation myths: Applying second language research to classroom teaching.* Ann Arbor: University of Michigan Press (pp. 188–234).

Saito, K., & Lyster, R. (2012). Effects of form-focused instruction and corrective feedback on L2 pronunciation development of /ɹ/ by Japanese learners of English. *Language Learning, 62*(2), 595–633.

Saito, K. 2012. Effects of instruction on L2 pronunciation development: A synthesis of 15 quasi-experimental intervention studies. *TESOL Quarterly, 46,* 842–854.

# 3

# Assessment

## Overview

Although there are vast differences in the world's languages, we expect all humans to acquire their mother tongue within similar timeframes through exposure beginning in the womb. We can identify milestones that appear to be near universals in terms of language development for all of the world's languages, but more importantly, we can track children's acquisition of individual languages, which allows us to establish clearly defined norms. If we measure any aspect of a child's language development and determine that it is significantly delayed in comparison to his or her typically-developing peers, we know that the child has a potential disorder, and we can take steps to determine possible interventions. In contrast, we do not generally have expectations or milestones for acquiring an L2, especially acquisition by adults. If two native English-speaking adults moved to China, and one learned to speak Mandarin relatively well after one year's time, and the other never developed basic communication skills within the same timeframe, we would not consider one of them to be normally developing and the other delayed or disordered. This basic fact helps us set the stage when assessing our non-native clients, since we must leave the concept of norms behind us right from the start. The purpose of our evaluation is not to determine how individuals compare to their peers, but rather to identify what aspects of clients' oral communication in their new language have the most significant impact on their ability to achieve their personal and professional goals. An effective second language oral communication assessment ascertains clients' attitudes and objectives, maps out their phonemic and phonotactic capabilities, identifies their suprasegmental strengths and weaknesses, and evaluates additional areas such as voice, fluency, language, or pragmatics that may interfere with communication. SLPs will therefore need to rely on a great deal of their training and expertise to conduct such assessments, but they will also need to step back at times to determine which aspects of a client's oral language are most likely to be salient to laypersons. Clinicians can balance impressionistic and objective judgments to identify how clients present at the beginning of training, and how to help them move forward.

## Purposes of Accent Assessments

In the film *Soldier of Orange* (Houwer & Verhoeven, 1977), which takes place in the Netherlands at the onset of the Second World War, there is a scene in which soldiers in the collapsing Dutch army fear that they have encountered a group of enemy combatants from Germany who are attempting to pass themselves off as speakers of Dutch. The soldiers ask the men they encounter to say the word *Scheveningen* because they know this will help them identify whether the combatants are native speakers or not. Forcing someone to speak in order to determine membership in a particular tribe goes back to the dawn of man. The word *shibboleth* refers to a word or belief that is used to identify group membership, and it comes from the biblical story in which the Gileadites identified and killed Ephraimites on the basis of their production of the initial /ʃ/ in that word (Block, Walton, Hess, & Manor, 2016). Similar stories throughout history and continuing to the modern day indicate that in some cases, testing for a particular accent can have extremely serious implications. Non-native speakers must sometimes pass an oral proficiency test to receive a degree, attain employment, or qualify for a license, for example, and issues related to intelligibility and accentedness may affect outcomes. Some of the most common tests of this type in the United States are the Test of Spoken English (TSE), the Test of English as a Foreign Language Internet based Test (TOEFL-IbT), and the Speaking Proficiency English Assessment Kit (SPEAK). There is also little doubt that informal assessments of accent are often used to determine whether someone gets a job or promotion.

In the world of TESOL, assessments are often divided into three types: needs assessments, summative assessments, and formative assessments. A needs assessment can determine a student's level to identify proper placement or to create goals for training. Summative assessments measure progress towards goals, and formative assessments provide evidence of outcomes. SLPs providing accent modification services use assessments for similar purposes as TESOL professionals. SLPs screen prospective clients in some way to determine whether services are appropriate, evaluate them to identify target areas, measure progress during training, and then conduct follow-up testing to document evidence of gains.

## Determining Clients' Goals

In maintaining a client-centered approach, it is important to take time to listen to clients and determine their personal goals concerning accent modification, keeping in mind that there may be a need to channel their motivations into realistic objectives. Despite the preponderance of evidence indicating the extreme rarity of attaining a native accent after puberty, it is relatively uncommon for a client to seek accent services with a good understanding of this fact. As discussed in Chapter 1, Derwing (2003) showed that 95% of those she surveyed wished to sound like a native speaker. Some clients specifically seek accent modification services with the stated goal of removing all traces of their accent, but many more may not mention this as their primary objective. Nevertheless, whether explicitly stated or not, many clients have a subconscious hope of never being asked where they are from again. During the assessment process, it is not important to address this issue head on, but it is helpful to lay the groundwork for future conversations and to identify personal goals that are more likely to be achievable during the sessions.

Often, the discussion of client objectives begins during the first stages of referral. Many initial contacts come through email or a third-party referral, and in most cases, these are followed up with discussion between clinician and client. Clinicians should focus carefully during these first conversations to determine a client's overall communication skills and the appropriacy of services. In some cases, clients may present with accentedness alone as opposed to any issues concerning intelligibility or naturalness, and it may be important to decline services and provide counseling on issues related to the critical period. There are ethical considerations involved in accepting clients who are unlikely to need fundamental changes in their communication skills. In other cases, clients may present with such significant difficulties in terms of intelligibility, syntax, vocabulary, or any other area of language use that training would be too challenging before the client attains higher second language proficiency. If there is no opportunity to have a direct conversation with the client, you can ask them to fill out an intake form, providing an opportunity for them to identify any personal goals they have related to accent.

A sample of the intake form used by San Diego State University's Accent and Communication Training Program (SDSU ACT Program) is included as Appendix 3–1 for adaptation and use. In designing this form, the goal was to create a simple document to provide the most relevant information related to accent. The form is relatively short compared to the clinic's general intake form, since there is no need to ask detailed questions related to health and background. Clients have an opportunity to describe any communication challenges they face in their native language to rule out any segmental or suprasegmental issues unrelated to second language phonological acquisition. It is unlikely that clients seeking accent modification services have a significant L1 communication disorder, but including a question about this gives them an opportunity to disclose it. Some practitioners may decide to test clients' hearing or conduct an oral motor examination to exclude any problems that might impact communication. The ACT program does not give clients an audiometric evaluation or any oral motor examinations out of a fear that clients may subconsciously perceive that accents are related to physiological abnormalities. Rather, the goal is to disassociate difference from disorder in clients' minds and to reassure them that it is normal to have an accent. In the rare case that a client has a hearing or oral motor issue that truly interferes with their ability to communicate, it is hoped that the client can determine this through interactions during the training itself.

Besides the personal information needed to contact the client, the most important sections of the intake form relate to native language, age of arrival, and self-rating of English proficiency in four different areas: pronunciation, listening, vocabulary, and grammar. As outlined in the section on the critical period hypothesis, age of arrival, or to be more precise, age of immersion, is the single best predictor of accent, and thus, it is the most valuable data point collected. Clients are also asked if they have had any previous accent training. Detailed information about clients' acquisition of English and experiences with accent modification can be solicited during discussions at a later date and can serve as good opportunities to acquire a spontaneous speech sample during the initial assessment, although many SLPs prefer to collect much of this information in writing before the client's first session. No matter how the information is collected, it is important to determine the client's use of English at work and home and to allow the client to elaborate on the contexts in which oral communication occurs in English throughout their day.

The assessment process itself is a perfect opportunity to document the client's individual objectives, simply by discussing this question. This conversation should also be reviewed as a part of a spontaneous language sample. If clients explicitly state that their goal is to sound exactly like a native speaker, they can be encouraged through follow-up questions to identify exactly how their oral communication interferes with their personal and professional goals, and this can be a good starting point to help build awareness about shifting the goal to effective communication. Separating personal and professional goals is beneficial because clients may have different preferences concerning these domains. The assessor should give clients free rein to discuss motivations since goals have a profound effect on the course of training. This is also an opportunity to offer some counseling, and most important of all, to lend a sympathetic ear to the client and establish rapport.

In addition to identifying personal goals, determining a client's attitudes and awareness can be an extremely effective way to establish baselines and to monitor the success of subsequent training. The ACT Attitude and Awareness Survey used at SDSU's Accent and Communication Training program is included as Appendix 3–2. In this survey, clients rate their agreement with statements according to a 5-point scale. Some of the statements are designed to gauge clients' attitudes about their accent (e.g., "It's very important for me to change the way I speak in English."), while others, such as, "I usually know where to put the stress on an English word," focus on awareness.

Clients read each statement aloud and then indicate their level of agreement using the scale. Although clients can also fill out this survey in advance, completing it together allows more opportunities for clarification and review. For example, the clinician can offer an example of intonation if the client is unsure what that term means. The survey provides a useful snapshot of clients' understanding of issues related to accentedness, intelligibility, and naturalness, and serves as a record of how they view their oral proficiency. At a later date, the survey can be readministered to provide objective evidence of clients' increased confidence and awareness.

## Segmental Assessment

In order for non-native speakers to produce intelligible speech, they need to produce accurate versions of all or most of the phonemes of their second language. A client who is not able to produce distinct versions of the vowels /i/ and /ɪ/ is likely to be frequently misunderstood. In addition, a substitution that is intelligible but not natural is likely to shift attention away from the client's message, as in the case of the substitution for the trilled /r/ for the American /ɹ/. Allophonic variations are also important, as in the case of clients who produce initial /p/ with too much or too little aspiration or use a /t/ where an American would use the alveolar tap. A segmental assessment allows clinicians to isolate the sounds of the language and determine which productions stray significantly from the native model. This type of assessment is often the most comfortable for SLPs entering the field of accent modification because it shares many commonalities with their experiences evaluating native-speaking children, with the notable exception that vowels receive the same amount of attention as consonants.

Following the principles of childhood articulation tests used for decades, the goal is to listen to the clients' productions of all or most of the key phonemes of the language in one or more positions. While children are generally shown a picture in order to elicit a target phoneme, adult clients are literate and can be prompted with written words. These words can be displayed on individual cards or in a list for the client to read. One practice not often used when working with native-speaking children, but which is common in the field of accent modification, is to have clients say a word once in isolation and then follow this up with an invented sentence using the word. The goal of the invented sentence is to provide an opportunity for a second, more spontaneous example of how the client might use the word in connected speech. Some published assessment measures in the field omit this step, but in many cases the target phoneme pronounced in isolation versus connected speech differ, and that can provide useful insight. Thus, a client given the word *dog* on a card with instructions to say the word by itself and then create a sentence using the word without altering it might say "dog, I took my dog for a walk." If clients change the word (e.g., adds an *s* and says "dogs"), they are prompted to try again without altering the word.

A good segmental assessment should include most (if not all) of the consonant and vowel phonemes of English, and the consonants should ideally be targeted in both initial and final position at a minimum. Two exceptions would be /ʒ, ŋ/. The /ʒ/ can be targeted intervocalically because it does not occur word initially and is relatively rare word finally, and the /ŋ/ can be targeted intervocalically or word finally since it also never occurs in initial position in English. The /t/ should also be targeted intervocalically to determine whether the client produces an alveolar tap allophonically. In a more extensive assessment, the other phonemes can be targeted intervocalically, but it may be more efficient to assess their production accuracy in the initial or final positions first. Some common consonant clusters and the major allophones of American English, such as the alveolar tap and syllabic /n/, should be included, and more in-depth assessments can add a wider variety of allophonic variations. The ACT Segmental Assessment used in SDSU's Accent and Communication Training program is included as Appendix 3–3, but clinicians are encouraged to develop their own sets of words. For a segmental assessment that uses a shorter list of words, see the Mini Accent Assessment, included as Appendix 3–4. While it is unlikely that an SLP would create their own version of a normed assessment of children's articulation, it is relatively straightforward to develop a good assessment tool crafted to a clinician's individual approach. In fact, a primary goal of this chapter is to give clinicians tips and tools for creating their own battery.

Clients should take a moment to review the assessment words before reading them aloud, and they can be encouraged to ask questions about their meaning and even their pronunciation. The primary goal of the segmental assessment is to determine the client's ability to produce the sounds of English, so clinicians should address any unfamiliarity with the pronunciation of the words due to the vagaries of English spelling. Clinicians should note the degree of clients' unfamiliarity with the words, to get an idea of their vocabulary level, but the focus should be on phonology. If a client misproduces a word during the assessment due to spelling interference, that is important to note, but the evaluation is not intended to gauge familiarity with orthography or vocabulary. At this point, on the ACT Segmental Assessment, clients can add four words to section B. Section B allows them to identify words that are difficult for them, which can save clinicians valuable time since the clients are often aware of particularly difficult segmentals or words which may be causing them significant difficulties in their daily lives. These words also offer clinicians a good opportunity to gauge intelligibility. The clinician should not view the words or ask about them until they are produced. The clinician should transcribe these words exactly as uttered and then later verify that the word was indeed the one intended by the client. If the clinician is unsure of the word as it is being produced, the client can be asked to repeat, explain, or even spell out the desired word.

Clinicians should record (with both audio and video if possible) the segmental assessment for later review. As is the case when conducting phonological assessments for children, pay close attention during the live productions and record notes as accurately as possible since this is the best opportunity to judge the accuracy of the phonemes, but having a backup is invaluable. Prior to the session, clinicians should transcribe the list of words comprising the segmental portion of the assessment on a scoresheet so that they can quickly make marks and notations without the need to transcribe the phonemes clients produce correctly. If the clinician misses a production, the client is asked to repeat it, or it can be rewiewed on the recording. In most cases, it is a worthwhile investment to review the recording for accuracy. Appendix 3–5 is a sample of the score sheet for the ACT Segmental Assessment.

Clinicians can make notes in much the same way they might when working with children's phonology. As a starting point, clinicians can use the SODA framework to identify substitutions, omissions, additions, and distortions. Substitutions, omissions, and additions can usually be notated by using slashes and identifying the added (or substituted) phoneme. For example, if a client produces the word *cave* as /keɪ/, the clinician can put a slash through the /v/. When identifying distortions, look for allophonic variations that deviate from native speaker norms; narrow transcription often provides an effective means of recording these differences. If the client fully devoices the /v/, the clinician can either cross out the /v/ and place an /f/ above or below it or use narrow transcription to indicate devoicing with a small circle below the phoneme /v̥/. Since voiced obstruents are normally somewhat devoiced in final position in English, using the devoicing symbol implies

**Table 3–1.** Useful IPA Diacritics for Assessment

| Diacritic | Meaning | Diacritic | Meaning |
|---|---|---|---|
| d̥ | devoiced/voiceless | æ̠ | Retracted |
| p̬ | voiced | a̟ | Advanced |
| æ̃ | nasalized | ʌ̞ | lowered |
| ŭ | extra short | ʌ̝ | raised |
| p˭ | unaspirated | i̹ | More rounded |
| pʰ | aspirated | u̜ | Less rounded |
| t̚ | no audible release | uː | lengthened |

that the phoneme was fully devoiced or sounded different than a typical production. Narrow transcription symbols are especially useful to note allophonic differences. In the same example, the clinician can mark the vowel with a diacritic if the client does not follow the rules of English phonology, which lengthens vowels before final voiced consonants. It is fairly common for clients to produce the word *cave* with a fully devoiced final /v/ and a shortened vowel, and this can be transcribed as [keɪ̆v̥]. To save time, clinicians do not need to add any diacritics to mark allophones produced correctly, so in this example, by not making a notation after the /k/, the implication is that the amount of aspiration produced was similar to the native model. If a client fails to produce aspiration, an additional diacritic could be added, and we would have [k˭eɪ̆v̥]. Table 3–1 lists several diacritics that are useful when working with accent clients. While the IPA is an efficient method to record clients' productions, and it can be readily interpreted by other professionals, clinicians are always welcome to use any system capable of marking these distinctions consistently and accurately.

Stimulability refers to the ability of a client to show immediate improvement following a short amount of modeling or training by the clinician. Clinicians can gauge stimulability either during or after the assessment by returning to troublesome segmentals and working with the client for a short amount of time to see if some progress can be made relatively quickly. Stimulability can play an important role in target selection, but it does not have to be evaluated during the initial assessment. In some cases, it may be preferable to determine the client's pure baseline before any training occurs.

In most cases, clinicians should take time to review the segmental assessment in detail to determine the client's phonemic inventory in English and identify any significant allophonic variations. Clinicians can review the results and map them out on a chart of the consonants and vowels. At this point, some phonotactic differences may emerge. For example, the client may have no difficulty producing voiced consonants word initially but may devoice them word finally. Other clients may delete final consonants that they produce accurately at the beginning of words. After a clear picture of the client's phonemic inventory and phonotactic differences from native speakers emerges, the clinician can move toward target selection.

## Intelligibility Assessment

One of the main goals of a second language phonological assessment is to determine the intelligibility of the non-native speaker's speech. Non-native speakers are essentially assessed on the clarity of their speech by their interlocutors in every communication exchange they engage in, and it is to some extent a part of each interaction they have with their clinician, beginning with their first discussion. Clinicians naturally begin to form general conclusions about the approximate intelligibility of a client's speech immediately, but it is helpful to use more objective measures. In many cases, it is sufficient to use clinical judgment to estimate the percentage of a client's speech that is intelligible, but estimates can be unreliable. Several studies have analyzed the connection between a listener's familiarity with particular L2 accents and their ability to understand speakers of that L2, and the results are inconsistent (see Carey, Mannell, & Dunn, 2011). But SLPs, especially those who spend a great deal of time working with non-native speakers, have a strong ability to compensate for variations in speech, and it can be difficult, therefore, to project the true intelligibility of a client when the L2 speaker communicates with untrained unfamiliar listeners. On a related note, there is some evidence for the logical notion that familiarity with a client leads to increased intelligibility (e.g., Bradlow & Bent, 2008; Kent, Miolo, & Bloedel, 1994), and this is important to keep in mind when assessing progress at a later date.

Some clinicians have used procedures designed for analyzing dysarthric speech, such as having clients read nonsense sentences that can be transcribed. The Sentence Intelligibility Test (Yorkston, Beukelman, & Tice, 1996). is a computer program that generates a series of random sentences that reduce the role of context in communicating ideas. An example sentence from the test, "For a different sort of tree, hang up colorful rolled up socks instead of ornaments," illustrates that speakers will need to produce the words *rolled up socks* clearly because listeners will not be expecting them (for other examples of such sentences see Nye & Gaitenby, 1974; and Picheny, Durlach, & Braida, 1985). Clinicians can print a list of these phrases and record the client saying them. Randomly generated sentences eliminate familiarity advantages when clinicians present clients with the sentences. Recordings can also be played for unfamiliar listeners. Clinicians can score intelligibility in several ways provided they maintain consistency when measuring progress. For example, a percentage of words identified correctly by a listener could be compared to the total number of words in the sentences. Another method scores only the content words to determine the percentage. This method offers a relatively objective way of determining intelligibility as long as clinicians keep several caveats in mind. First, this approach uses the narrow definition of the term intelligibility—that is, the ability to convey phonemes, words, and sentences accurately—but it may not provide a complete description of a non-native speaker's ability to convey a message as a whole. In some cases, a client may be able to convey the overall meaning successfully even when some individual sounds or words are not identified accurately by the listener, while in other cases, the sounds or words may be accurate, but problems with suprasegmentals or naturalness may interfere with communication. Second, the clinician must be careful when using this method to demonstrate progress, since intelligibility automatically increases due to familiarity.

Another method of gauging intelligibility is to use a series of true/false statements that involve basic knowledge, such as "whales are large animals that live in the ocean." The client can read and record the series of statements, and an unfamiliar listener can mark them as true or false. The assumption is that any statements marked incorrectly would be the result of intelligibility issues. In theory, a large number of these could be produced and randomly printed for the clinician to score, but in practice, it is probably easiest to use untrained, unfamiliar listeners.

A recent study (Kang, Thomson, & Moran, 2018) reviewed five different means of measuring intelligibility, including several of the methods just discussed, to evaluate their relative efficacy, primarily with regard to how they might predict a non-native speaker's ability to understand someone. The methods discussed included some that could be useful for research but are probably less practical for L2 phonological assessments, such as the use of low-pass filtering of words in a transcription task, a cloze transcription exercise in which some words are provided in advance to the listeners, and the use of scalar judgments. The authors advised practitioners to experiment with different types of intelligibility measures depending on the intended goal and to combine them with an examination of the segmental and suprasegmental features of non-native speech. There is clearly a need to continue developing accurate measures that are easy to administer. Developments in automated speech recognition will most likely allow future evaluations to gauge some aspects of pronunciation without involving a human listener. Some electronic assessments have already been marketed in the ESL community, but mainly as a way to screen the pronunciation of large groups of students, and it is unlikely that they would be useful for SLPs working with individual clients or small groups.

## Suprasegmental Assessment

Suprasegmentals can be assessed in several ways, ranging from evaluation of single words to scoring lengthy speech samples. Typical methods involve having clients read words or phrases, respond to prompts, listen to and evaluate sentences, read a diagnostic passage aloud, or produce a spontaneous speech sample. It is somewhat artificial to separate suprasegmentals out since SLPs should be focused on all aspects of speech, such as stress, intonation, phrasing, rate, voice, and breath support, during every step of the assessment process, but the procedures below are intended to focus primarily on aspects of speech at this level.

Suprasegmental features such as word and phrasal stress, intonation, and linking can be assessed by having clients read a word or sentence from a sheet of prompts, either in isolation or in response to a statement or question. Even during segmental assessments, any multisyllabic words offer clues to the client's ability to produce stress on the correct syllable and in a natural way. If the SLP wants more detailed information about the client's ability to produce lexical stress, words with alternating stress can be used. For example, the clinician can ask the client to read aloud a series of words such as *photograph, photography, photographic*, which will provide valuable information about naturalness and accuracy of stress, as well as expose vowel reductions and allophonic variations. Words with stress shifts depending on parts of speech (e.g., *record* as a verb vs. *record* as a noun) can be targeted in a similar way. A client's ability to produce appropriate phrasal stress can be assessed through short sentences read aloud, although this may be easier to target in lengthier passages. SLPs can test intonation and emphasis discretely by asking clients to read written prompts in response to a question or statement. For example, intonation could be tested by giving the client a prompt as simple as the basic exclamation *oh* and then asking them to say it in response to a statement such as "I had a flat tire this morning" or "Dave just won the lottery." In some published accent modification assessment materials, clients are asked a question or given a statement to which they respond by reading a word or phrase. For example, the clinician might ask "Where did she go?" and the client would read the response "She went to the store." The clinician's scoresheet would have a visual representation of the expected pitch contour for the sentence, and the clinician can judge the response according to how accurately it aligned with expectations. One possible risk to this approach is that deviation from the perceived contour may not correlate with naturalness ratings by native speakers. In other words, the visual representation of the expected contour may not be sufficient to represent the range of possible prosodic patterns that would be deemed acceptable by listeners. Although the desire to create more objective measurements of suprasegmentals is understandable, clinicians are probably best served by relying on their own judgment of appropriateness since there is such a wide range of possible patterns. Suprasegmentals can also be assessed through perception tasks. For example, clients might be asked to determine a speaker's intention or attitude after listening to statements read with various intonation patterns.

To test emphasis, a client might be given the prompt, "She's in the bathroom," and then asked the question "Is she outside the bathroom?" to determine whether they can correctly put the stress on the preposition in the response. Linking can be evaluated by having clients read sentences such as, "That is what I can eat after I run a lot" to assess the intervocalic connections and allophonic variations.

## Diagnostic Passages

The use of a diagnostic passage is another method commonly used to assess suprasegmentals, and it will also provide useful information about segmentals, especially in terms of allophones. Typically, a client is asked to read the passage through silently once or twice to prepare, and when ready, the clinician takes notes while the client reads through the text. One of the principal advantages of this type of assessment is that it allows clinicians to hear clients engage in a lengthier sample of discourse, and this provides better opportunities to analyze suprasegmental features such as intonation, linking, phrasal stress, and emphasis. Passages are also an easy way to measure rate since clinicians can collect data from native and non-native speakers on the same text. This saves considerable time because the number of words or syllables can be counted in advance and then used as a reference for all future clients. See Chapter 5 for a discussion of how to calculate appropriate rates, but as a ballpark number, look for ranges between about 120 and 260 words per minute. Regardless of the actual number of words or syllables per minute, it is important to use clinical judgment to determine whether the rate of speech sounds excessively slow, natural, or too rapid. Once again, the numbers are merely guidelines since perception is key. The passage can contain words with variable stress to determine clients' awareness of stress in English. The word *record* can be used as both a noun and a verb in the same passage, for example, to ascertain whether a client understands the rules governing the stress of this word.

A well-constructed diagnostic passage can also provide more information about clients' segmentals, especially in terms of allophonic variation and coarticulation. For example, a sentence containing a phrase such as "but it is" could be used to determine whether the client uses an alveolar tap when linking words in connected speech. These texts are usually designed to provide good opportunities to hear most (if not all) of the phonemes of American English. In short, diagnostic passages are an efficient way to hear some important segmental and suprasegmental features of English that might take much longer to elicit through spontaneous speech. The passage can also be repeated at a later time to measure progress, and in that case, it is helpful to discuss the client's increased awareness following training, even when some of the productions may be similar to what they were before training.

The primary disadvantage of diagnostic passages is that it is often difficult to separate pronunciation errors from errors due to unfamiliarity with the words in the text. In addition, diagnostic passages may be less useful for determining intelligibility because clinicians hear them repeatedly and will have a much more difficult time disassociating their own familiarity with the text from clients' production. Finally, clients perform differently when they use words in their active vocabulary, as opposed to words they may use rarely, if ever. These passages are also less related to clients' real world needs since they are less likely to be reading aloud than speaking. Clinicians should always work with clients to determine how they use English in their personal and professional lives, but it is generally uncommon for clients to need to read aloud texts that they have not written themselves or had time to review.

Although the field of speech-language pathology has a tradition of using texts such as the "Rainbow Passage," and the "Grandfather Passage," these are probably less suitable for non-native speaking clients. In the "Rainbow Passage," for example, phrases such as, "these take the shape of a long round arch, with its path high above, and its two ends apparently beyond the horizon," may require some additional processing time for speakers whose L1 is not English. Moreover, the "Grandfather Passage" features low frequency words such as *zest, frock, utmost* and *quiver,* and there is little chance that non-natives are familiar with *banana oil* since native speakers rarely are. The International Speech Accent Archive does, however, have many samples of non-native speakers reading the "Rainbow Passage" as well as "Comma Gets a Cure" and "Please Call Stella." The latter two passages were created for the site and can be found at the archive or through an internet search. "Please Call Stella" is relatively short at just 69 words, while the full version of "Comma Gets a Cure" has 375 words. Both of them feature modern, relatively colloquial English. Another option is the recently published "Caterpillar Passage" (Patel, Connaghan, Franco, Edsall, Forgit, Olsen, & Russell, 2013), which contains 196 words and was designed for the assessment of motor speech disorders. Typical diagnostic passages range from 100 to 200 words, and the diagnostic passage from SDSU's Accent and Communication Training program included here as Appendix 3–6 contains 149 words. A passage much shorter than 100 words is unlikely to provide enough opportunity to evaluate segmental and suprasegmental information, and anything much longer than 200 words would probably tax the client.

## Spontaneous Speech Sample

There will almost always be some type of spontaneous speech sample during the initial referral and screening process or initial evaluation since the SLP and client will interact and engage in conversation. It is also beneficial to set aside some part of the session for the SLP to ask clients questions more formally, or provide prompts to elicit a longer sample. SLPs can undoubtedly benefit from analyzing a combination of both overtly- and covertly- collected speech samples. In other words, during some sections of the assessment the client is informed that a speech sample is being collected, and there are also opportunities for off the cuff interactions that can provide valuable insights into how the client speaks when focused more on content than form. SLPs should keep in mind that simple gestures such as jotting something down on a clipboard will elevate the client's awareness of the evaluation process, so at times it may be useful to make mental notes and then refer back to recordings during some of these more candid moments of conversation.

When eliciting speech samples, SLPs can ask broad questions about clients' personal or professional life or focus more narrowly on their experiences acquiring or using English. To save time, collect these samples as part of the process of determining clients' needs. Such opportunities are a valuable way to glimpse clients' ability to communicate naturally about subjects they are familiar with while allowing them the greatest freedom for word selection. It is generally a good idea to begin the assessment with these types of activities since they help establish rapport and ease clients into more structured activities that may make them more cautious. If possible, clinicians should make audiovisual recordings of these spontaneous samples, and if clients are asked to bring in recordings of responses to prompts, it's important to make sure clients do not practice their responses in advance since spontaneity is of key import. It is usually easy to ascertain that someone is reading something as opposed to speaking spontaneously, and it is especially obvious when clients are not as proficient in English. Non-native speakers' performances on reading aloud tasks versus spontaneous speech show differences in error patterns (Levis & Barriuso,

2012). Since SLPs benefit from having a look at the widest range of communication, best practice would appear to be a combination of spontaneous and rehearsed speech.

# Assessing Pragmatics

During all stages of assessment, and from the first moment of client contact, SLPs should focus on how the client's pragmatics affect their communication. Most SLPs have excellent training and backgrounds in pragmatics; it is second nature for them to pay close attention to eye contact, proxemics, conversational balance, topic maintenance, along with countless other aspects of communication that shape a client's ability to interact with listeners effectively. When working with clients from other countries and cultures, they can add to this list by also focusing on facial expressions and gestures that may stand out in comparison to cultural norms, These aspects can be particularly challenging for non-native speaking clients, who have typically been conditioned by their societies for many years to use pragmatics that may seem alien in other environments. Clients from certain cultures may present with flat affect because it is the cultural norm in conversations not involving family members or friends, while others may falsely convey elation or agitation. Since SLPs are trained to respect other cultures and communication styles, they may have to step back and consider how these differences may cause miscommunication for interlocutors not expecting them.

An excellent way to supplement the information obtained by observing clients throughout the assessment is to use role plays that give clients more structured opportunities to use all aspects of communication. Role plays can range from simply asking the client to pretend to be in a social situation or interview to more elaborate situations such as having the client ask for a raise or resolve a misunderstanding politely. Appendix 3–7 offers some sample role play prompts. Providing a variety of contexts allows clinicians to see if a client might be appropriately friendly and engaging in a social situation but then appear overly casual in a mock interview. Clinicians should record these interactions on video for later review to identify potential problems, focusing on identifying any behavior that would tend to shift the focus from what clients are saying to how they are communicating it.

# Evaluating Through Listening and Writing

Clinicians may wish to consider some type of listening or writing task, but the risk is that there may not be a strong correlation between the results from this type of evaluation and the client's ability to produce clear and natural speech. Some larger programs in the world of TESOL have attempted to use written assessments, but evidence suggests that this type of testing is ineffective (Buck, 1989). These tests generally involve tasks such as identifying which words in a group are pronounced with the same sounds. For example, examinees are given the word *least* as a prompt and have to determine which word from the set of *great*, *steak*, *bread*, *pleasure*, and *cease* has the same vowel sound. Awareness of stress can be tested in writing as well, by asking clients to identify which words fit a stress pattern or have a stress shift. Since SLPs are generally not interested in screening large numbers of potential clients, this type of testing may be of limited value because of its strong connection to orthographic awareness and its poor ability to predict a client's actual oral proficiency. SLPs can collect some type of writing sample to get additional insight into clients' overall English language abilities, especially if they are planning to work on grammar or language use during their sessions, but otherwise these tests are of limited value in assessing L2 phonology.

At the segmental level, perceptual testing can involve listening discrimination, in which clients are asked to determine whether words have the same or different vowel or consonant sounds, or to identify which word they hear from a list of minimal pairs or sets. To test suprasegmentals, clinicians can have clients identify which syllable is stressed after listening to a model of a word, or which word is stressed after listening to a model of a sentence using emphatic stress. Although some perceptual testing asks clients to identify whether sentences have rising or falling intonation patterns, even native speakers may have difficulty making this type of determination, so they are unlikely to indicate clients' ability to imitate or spontaneously produce these patterns accurately. A client's understanding of features related to spontaneous, reduced speech can be evaluated by having them fill in missing function words in rapidly spoken natural sentences. Overall, while perceptual testing can provide some useful information, it is best suited for screening large groups of non-natives, which is much more likely to occur in the TESOL context as opposed to accent modification conducted by SLPs. As noted above, if an SLP intends to work on all aspects of communication in English, then it is certainly important to measure listening comprehension, but if the focus is on speech, then a client's perception will have less value than their production.

## Evaluating Language

To this point, we have not discussed how to assess  the syntax and vocabulary of clients' language. While there is no doubt that these play a huge role in communication, there are various viewpoints on the need to evaluate them. From the discussion on the critical period hypothesis, it is evident that there are different expectations for ultimate attainment when comparing phonology to other linguistic areas such as syntax or semantics. While we do not expect non-native speaking clients to achieve native accents, it is certainly possible (and indeed not uncommon) for non-native speakers to attain grammaticality judgment abilities and vocabularies that are on par with natives or even surpass them. In addition, SLPs tend to focus on oral communication and leave English language teaching to TESOL instructors. Some SLPs working in accent modification focus entirely on clients' phonology, and some may even work only with clients who have near-native syntax and vocabulary.

To some extent, there will be a grammar and vocabulary component of any accent assessment that goes beyond a simple segmental evaluation. SLPs should always keep tabs on a client's overall language level and their ability to construct syntactically accurate sentences with appropriate vocabulary. In all cases it is important to develop an understanding of the relationship between a client's broader abilities in English and their pronunciation. Speech-language pathologists working in accent modification tend to seek out clients whose phonological abilities are significantly lower than their abilities in the other realms of language, and often feel that clients with low overall levels of English can benefit more from focusing on other aspects of the language before seeking help with pronunciation. Those who choose to focus on developing a client's overall language skills may wish to evaluate grammar, vocabulary, or perhaps writing in detail. The TESOL field has many tests available that can be adapted for these purposes. However, for most SLPs, an informal review of the client's English during spontaneous speech should suffice.

## Assessment Packages

Many clinicians use informal measures to determine appropriate goals for working on accent with their non-native clients, and sometimes assessments used in other areas of our field are adapted for second language phonology. Tests designed for working with dysarthric clients can be easily adapted for accent modification, including the Sentence Intelligibility Test mentioned above, and the Assessment of Intelligibility of Dysarthric Speech (Yorkston, Beukelman, & Traynor, 1981). In contrast, materials for testing L1 phonology are rarely used because they are designed for children and based on a developmental framework. One goal of this book is to empower clinicians to develop an evaluation process that leads to the best results for clients, and Appendix 3–8 lists several frameworks to help adapt the ideas and examples provided here. There are also commercially available assessments specifically designed for accent modification, which have several advantages. They can save a considerable amount of time since they do not require the clinician to invest count-less hours developing a comprehensive assessment, although in some cases they may require training to learn how to administer them. In addition, since they are used by other clinicians around the world, there is more data available for comparisons. They also look professional and attractive to clients, and they may be one part of a series of materials available for purchase. The following are several noteworthy examples, although there may be other excellent sets not mentioned here.

The Pronouncing English as a Second Language (PESL) Screening and Phonological Assessment (Compton, 2002) is based on the Pronouncing English as a Second Language method developed by Arthur J. Compton in 1980. This program, often referred to simply as "Compton," has been on the market the longest and is perhaps the best known among SLPs. The test has an online version that allows SLPs who have been trained in their program to administer the assessment and score it electronically. Clients take the test online, and the recordings can be reviewed and scored afterwards by the clinician. The assessment consists of four sections focusing on the segmental level of speech production. In the first section, clients read 30 stimulus words in isolation and then in a sentence of their choice, and in the next section they read a diagnostic passage. The 3rd section consists of a modeled reading section in which the client reads along silently while listening to a sentence and then repeats it. In the final section, clients produce a spontaneous speech sample in response to prompts. When the assessment is complete, an SLP analyzes the segmentals to determine which sounds are omitted, added, or substituted. There are specific scoring sheets for each language, which makes analysis easier because anticipated errors are listed next to the model and can be clicked on easily. Any errors that stray from these expectations can be added using IPA symbols, and clinicians can make notes as well. Although the test does not evaluate suprasegmentals, clinicians are asked to note any grammatical errors. The program also creates a personalized report, identifying segmental error patterns.

The Comprehensive Assessment of Accentedness & Intelligibility (CAAI) was developed by Amee Shah in 2007 as a more objective way to assess accented speech. The test is comprehensive in that it evaluates many areas related to accentedness and intelligibility. Clients receive numerical scores, which allows clinicians to establish clear baselines and assess progress. The results indicate the client's severity of communication difficulties, which provides an objective measure of a client's oral proficiency in English and can be used to create training programs. The CAAI is currently in use in over 172 universities and speech and hearing clinics and there are opportunities to share data for research. According to the developer, the complete assessment takes approximately one hour, but clinicians can select which of the 22 sections to administer based on the level and needs of the client. The test is divided into four main sections: baseline intelligibility and rate of speech, speech production abilities, speech perception, and language.

In keeping with research related to separating accentedness from intelligibility, the assessment requires clinicians to rate the accentedness of clients reading individual sentences before they read the "Rainbow Passage" to gauge intelligibility. In the speech production section, clinicians examine segmentals, suprasegmentals, and phonological patterns. To assess intonation, clients read words and phrases in response to statements or questions, and clinicians determine whether the pitch contour matched a suggested norm. Non-native speakers' ability to produce accurate lexical stress in different types of words (i.e., words with derivative or contrastive stress) is measured by having clients read a specific word aloud in response to questions, or by having them read various words or sentences provided to them on a prompt sheet. The battery evaluates a variety of other suprasegmental features of English as well, and targets segmentals by having clients read lists of words in isolation. Phonological processes are assessed in a subtest that has clients read target sentences geared toward identifying typical non-native patterns. In the speech perception section, auditory discrimination tests require the client to determine whether two words in a pair are the same or different or to write down the exact word they hear. Lastly, the language subtests focus on clients' understanding of idiomatic expressions, syntax, and vocabulary, as well as pragmatics, such as facial expressions, gestures, and topic initiation. Clinicians score each section of the test and assign a rating based on normative percentages, This also allows the test to serve as an objective measure of progress following training. The test kit includes protocols, intake forms, scoring guides, and a sample report.

The 7th edition of the Proficiency in Oral English Communication (POEC) (Sikorski, 2018) is available in paper and electronic formats and consists of seven subtests that can be administered in approximately one hour. Subtest I allows clinicians to establish rapport while also monitoring carefully for pragmatics and overall English oral proficiency. The clinician asks personal background questions and makes notations on the scoresheet concerning language use, pragmatics, and any significant phonemic or suprasegmental errors. Subtest II has the clients read prompts in response to questions or statements, and clinicians match the responses to diagrams of the words' lexical stress pattern. Subtest III is similar, but the client reads phrases and clinicians compare them to an expected pitch contour diagramed above each phrase on the scoresheet. Subtest IV focuses on segmentals; clients read a prompt in isolation and then create a sentence containing the word. Subtest V assesses clients' ability to use appropriate stress by emphasizing the correct word in a sentence in response to specific questions asked by the clinician. Section VI is an auditory discrimination task in which clients listen to two words and determine whether they are the same or different. Spontaneous speech samples are collected in Section VII, which is supplemental and has several optional tasks that give the client a chance to converse with the clinician or with other individuals.

The Clearspeak Adult Pronunciation (CAP) Test (Kimble-Fry, 2004) is a qualitative assessment tool developed by Alison Kimble-Fry primarily for use in Australia, but it can be adapted for use in any English-speaking country. The test consists of five subtests focusing on vowels, consonants, and prosody. The first subtest is designed to assess overall speech quality with a short diagnostic passage that the client reads aloud. The passage provides opportunities to hear clients produce English phonemes and allows clinicians to assess suprasegmental features as well. In the second subtest (Sentences for Vowels and Diphthongs) clients read 17 sentences containing the vowels and diphthongs of English aloud, and in the third subtest (Sentences for Consonants), seven sections, comprising five sentences each, target consonants. The sections are organized into sentences that contrast specific consonant phonemes. The fourth subtest (Stress Patterns in Words) consists of sets of words that tend to give non-native speakers difficulty in terms of lexical stress. The words in each set are homophonic or share a root. For example clients may be asked to read "economic, economy, economical" in order to determine their ability to shift the stress appropriately. In the final section, clients speak for one minute on a subject of their choice to provide information about suprasegmentals. A shorter version of the test, which can be used as a screener, is included in Alison Kimble-Fry's book (2001). It contains shorter versions of the first three subtests and a speech sample reading passage, but it does not independently assess lexical stress.

# Final Thoughts

Assessment can appear to be one of the most challenging aspects for SLPs working in the field of accent modification. When working with clients who have disabilities, SLPs understand that formal assessment instruments provide just one piece of an elaborate puzzle, and the results always need to be interpreted in conjunction with a host of other factors. SLPs working in the field of accent modification can use their backgrounds as communication experts and their unique ability to identify clients' true communication skills to craft creative assessments that paint a detailed portrait of clients' oral proficiency in English. It may take some extra work and planning, but it is well within reach, and the investment in time and effort during this initial process pays for itself in results during training.

# References

Block, D. I., Walton, J. H., Hess, R., & Manor, D. W. (2016). *Joshua, Judges, and Ruth.* Grand Rapids, MI: Zondervan.

Bradlow, A. R., & Bent, T. (2008). Perceptual adaptation to non-native speech. *Cognition, 106,* 707–729.

Buck, G. (1989). Written tests of pronunciation: Do they work? *ELT Journal, 43*(1), 50–56.

Carey, M., Mannell, R., & Dunn, P. (2011). Does a rater's familiarity with a candidate's pronunciation affect the rating in oral proficiency interviews? *Language Testing, 28*(2), 201–219.

Compton, A. (2002), *Pronouncing English as a Second Language (PESL) Screening and Phonological Assessment* [Assessment instrument]. San Francisco, CA: Carousel House Press.

Derwing, T. (2003). What do ESL students say about their accents? *Canadian Modern Language Review, 59*(4), 547–566.

Derwing, T. M., & Munro, M. J. (2015). *Pronunciation fundamentals: Evidence-based perspectives for L2 teaching and research.* Amsterdam, The Netherlands: John Benjamins.

Houwer, R. (Producer), & Verhoeven, P. (Director). (1977). *Soldaat van Oranje/Soldier of Orange* [Motion picture]. The Netherlands: Excelsior Films.

Kang, O., Thomson, R., & Moran, M. (2018). Empirical approaches to measuring the intelligibility of different varieties of English in predicting listener comprehension. *Language Learning, 68*(1), 115–146.

Kent, R. D., Miolo, G., & Bloedel, S. (1994). The intelligibility of children's speech: A review of evaluation procedures. *American Journal of Speech-Language Pathology, 3,* 81–95

Kimble-Fry, A., & ClearSpeak (2001). *Perfect pronunciation: A guide for trainers and self-help students.* Sydney, Australia: ClearSpeak Pty Ltd.

Kimble-Fry, A., & ClearSpeak (2004). *Clearspeak Adult Pronunciation (CAP) test* [Assessment Instrument]. Sydney, Australia: ClearSpeak Pty Ltd.

Levis, J., & Barriuso, T. (2012). Segmental errors in conversational and read speech: A comparison of ESL learners from four language backgrounds. In J. Levis & K. LeVelle (Eds.), *Proceedings of the 3rd Pronunciation in Second Language Learning and Teaching Conference* (pp. 187–194), Ames, IA: Iowa State University.

Nye, P. W., & Gaitenby, J. H. (1974). The intelligibility of synthetic monosyllabic words in short, syntactically normal sentences. *Haskins Laboratories Status Report in Speech Research. SR-37/38,* 169–190.

Patel, R., Connaghan, K., Franco, D., Edsall, E., Forgit, D., Olsen, L., & Russell, S. (2013). "The caterpillar": a novel reading passage for assessment of motor speech disorders. *American Journal of Speech Language Pathology / American Speech Language Hearing Association, 22*(1), 1–9.

Picheny M., Durlach N., & Braida L. (1985). Speaking clearly for the hard of hearing I: Intelligibility differences between clear and conversational speech. *Journal of Speech and Hearing Research 28,* 96–103.

Shah, A. P. (2007). *Comprehensive Assessment of Accentedness Intelligibility (CAAI)* [Assessment instrument]. Cleveland, OH: EBAM Institute.

Sikorski, L. (2018). *Proficiency in Oral English Communication (POEC).* [Assessment instrument]. Santa Ana, CA: LDS & Associates.

Yorkston, K., Beukelman, D., & Traynor, C. (1981). *Assessment of Intelligibility of Dysarthric Speech* [Assessment instrument]. Austin, TX: Pro-Ed.

Yorkston, K., Beukelman, D. R., & Tice, R. (1996). *Sentence Intelligibility Test* [Assessment instrument]. Lincoln, NE: Tice Technologies.

# 3-1

# Sample Intake Form

**University Speech-Language Clinic**

**Address**

**Phone**

**Email**

## Initial Application Form—Accent and Communication Training (ACT)

Date of Application _____ Please check one: ☐ Student ☐ Faculty ☐ Community Member

1. Sessions are _____. Are you available at those times? ☐ Yes ☐ No

2. First name _____ Last name _____

3. Date of birth _____ Age _____ Gender _____

4. Address _____

5. Preferred phone _____ Alternate phone _____

6. Email _____

7. How did you find out about the program? _____

8. Language you speak best _____ Other language(s) you know _____

9. Age of arrival in the US _____ Country of birth _____

10. Other countries you have lived in _____

11. Highest level of education _____

12. Employer/job title: _____

13. Please rate your English in the following areas on a scale from 1–10 (1 = absolute beginner, 10 = near native)

    Pronunciation _____      Grammar _____

    Vocabulary _____      Comprehension _____

14. Have you ever had English accent training? ☐ Yes ☐ No
    If yes, please describe:

15. Do you have any significant communication problems in your native language? If yes, please explain.

16. Is there other information we should know about your medical, social, or communication history?

    Any questions?

    Clinic Email: _____ Clinic Phone: _____

# 3-2

# ACT Attitude and Awareness Survey

Name:

Date:

| strongly disagree | disagree | not sure | agree | strongly agree |
|---|---|---|---|---|
| 1 | 2 | 3 | 4 | 5 |

| Statement | Score |
|---|---|
| It's very important for me to change the way I speak English. | |
| I am an effective communicator in English. | |
| My English pronunciation is clear. | |
| My English pronunciation is natural. | |
| I am often nervous when speaking because of my pronunciation. | |
| My English pronunciation causes me problems. | |
| I have a good understanding of English speech sounds. | |
| I have a good awareness of English intonation and speech patterns. | |
| My pronunciation is not as good as my other abilities in English. | |
| People often have difficulty understanding me because of my accent. | |

| I understand the English vowel system. | |
|---|---|
| I have good knowledge of the consonants of English. | |
| Most non-native speakers have better pronunciation than I do. | |
| I usually know where to put the stress on English words. | |
| I feel good about my accent in English. | |

# ACT Segmental Assessment

**A. Read aloud each word once and then use it in a sentence. Remember not to change the word.**

Example: *"house" I want to buy a house.*

| | |
|---|---|
| 1. fish | 15. gap |
| 2. judge | 16. dig |
| 3. Tom | 17. pet |
| 4. ride | 18. voice |
| 5. thing | 19. there |
| 6. mouth | 20. weather |
| 7. safe | 21. pleasure |
| 8. nail | 22. yet |
| 9. cave | 23. singer |
| 10. book | 24. potato |
| 11. shoes | 25. heater |
| 12. zone | 26. stars |
| 13. lab | 27. world |
| 14. church | 28. certain |

**B. Choose four words that are difficult for you to pronounce. Say each word alone, and then say it in a sentence.**

1. _____

2. _____

3. _____

4. _____

# 3-4

# Mini Accent Assessment

**1. Interview**

**2. Read aloud the following passage:**

Although children can easily learn to speak a second language with a native accent, adults are not as fortunate. Every language has different sounds and speaking patterns, and learners have to readjust their mouths and minds in order to adapt. The following are some useful tips for improving your pronunciation. First, familiarize yourself with the sounds of the new language. Don't worry about how the words are written; trust your ears and not your eyes. If a certain sound is hard to make, work until you get it right. Second, talk to native speakers or record their voices, listening closely to their intonation, phrasing, and stress. Finally, keep a record of your progress to help you stay motivated and focused. Keep in mind that the path to learning to speak a second language with a clear and natural accent can be difficult, but it is well worth the effort.

**3. Mini screening assessment**

Read aloud each word once and then use it in a sentence. Don't change the word.

Example: *"house" I want to buy a house in San Diego.*

| | | |
|---|---|---|
| third | shoes | teeth |
| scratch | blocks | buddy |
| other | zipper | chair |
| horse | judge | look |
| spring | witch | ring |

**4. Spontaneous Speech Sample** (Ask about a typical day, a good vacation, a hobby, etc.)

# 3–5

# ACT Segmental Assessment Score Sheet

**A. Read each word once and then use it in a sentence. Remember not to change the word (e.g., houses instead of house).**

Example: *"house" I want to buy a house.*

1. fish /fɪʃ/
2. judge /dʒʌdʒ/
3. Tom /tɑm/
4. ride /ɹaɪd/
5. thing /θɪŋ/
6. mouth /maʊθ/
7. safe /seɪf/
8. nail /neɪl/
9. cave /keɪv/
10. book /bʊk/
11. shoes /ʃuz/
12. zone /zoʊn/
13. lab /læb/
14. church /tʃɝtʃ/
15. gap /gæp/
16. dig /dɪg/
17. pet /pɛt/
18. voice /vɔɪs/
19. there /ðɛɚ/
20. weather /wɛðɚ/
21. pleasure /plɛʒɚ/
22. yet /jɛt/
23. singer /sɪŋɚ/
24. potato /pəteɪɾoʊ/
25. heater /hiɾɚ/
26. stars /stɑɚz/
27. world /wɝld/
28. certain /sɝʔn̩/

**B. Choose four words that are difficult for you to pronounce. Say each word alone, and then say it in a sentence.**

1. _____   2. _____

3. _____   4. _____

Scoring

## Consonants

| | Initial | Final | | Initial | Final |
|---|---|---|---|---|---|
| p | | | ʃ | | |
| t | | | ʧ | | |
| k | | | ʤ | | |
| b | | | l | | |
| d | | | ɹ | | |
| g | | | m | | |
| f | | | n | | |
| v | | | | Medial | Final |
| s | | | ŋ | | |
| z | | | ʒ | | |
| θ | | | | Initial | Final |
| | Initial | Medial | w | | |
| ð | | | j | | |
| ɾ | | | h | | |

## Clusters/Syllabic /n/

| | Initial | Final |
|---|---|---|
| pl | | |
| st | | |
| ɚld | | |
| n̩ | | |

## Words

| | |
|---|---|
| | |
| | |
| | |
| | |

## Vowels

| i | | ɪ | |
|---|---|---|---|
| eɪ | | ɛ | |
| æ | | ɑ | |
| ʌ | | ɝ | |
| ə | | ɚ | |
| u | | ʊ | |
| oʊ | | aɪ | |
| aʊ | | ɔɪ | |

# 3-6

# ACT Diagnostic Passage

Although children can easily learn to speak a second language with a native accent, adults are not as fortunate. Every language has different sounds and speaking patterns, and learners have to readjust their mouths and minds in order to adapt. The following are some useful tips for improving your pronunciation. First, familiarize yourself with the sounds of the new language. Don't worry about how the words are written; trust your ears and not your eyes. If a certain sound is hard to make, work until you get it right. Second, talk to native speakers or record their voices, listening closely to their intonation, phrasing, and stress. Finally, keep a record of your progress to help you stay motivated and focused. Keep in mind that the path to learning to speak a second language with a clear and natural accent can be difficult, but it is well worth the effort.

# 3-7

# Sample Role Play Prompts

| | |
|---|---|
| I was hired by your company to cut costs, and I called you in to discuss your job. Explain to me what you do, and why you are necessary for the company. | You and I are friends. I want to stay home, and you want to go out to do something. Try to convince me. |
| You are my best friend. I decided to get married, but you think I'm making a big mistake. Explain to me why I shouldn't get married. | Your company would like to give you a promotion, but they want you to explain all of the changes you would make once you start your new position. |
| I am thinking about having the same job that you do. Tell me why you think that's a good or bad idea. What are all of the advantages and disadvantages of your position? | You are my neighbor, and you don't like living next door to me because a lot of things I do bother you. Tell me about the problems I'm causing. |

# Sample Assessment Outlines

**Phone Screening (5 minutes)**

1. Interview about needs
   - Where and when client speaks English
   - Any significant personal/professional problems related to accent
   - Goals
2. Spontaneous language sample. This may be unnecessary if the client has had enough opportunities to speak at length during the interview. Otherwise use a basic prompt, such as, "tell me about yourself, family, job, hobbies," etc.

**Mini Assessment (15 minutes)**

1. Short interview
   - Where and when client speaks English
   - Any significant personal/professional problems related to accent
   - Goals
2. Diagnostic passage (50–200 words)
   - "Please Call Stella," "Comma Gets a Cure," "Rainbow Passage," ACT Diagnostic passage, etc.
3. Short segmental assessment of words
   - 10–15 words (see sample screener)
4. Spontaneous speech sample

**Standard Assessment (45 minutes–1 hour)**

1. Interview
   - Where and when client speaks English

- Any significant personal/professional problems related to accent
- Questions about personal and professional life
- Goals

2. Diagnostic passage (50–200 words)
   - Please Call Stella, Comma Gets a Cure, Rainbow Passage, ACT diagnostic passage, etc.
3. Segmental assessment of all consonant and vowel phonemes
   - 15–30 words and sentences (see sample)
4. Spontaneous speech sample
   - Prompts related to personal/professional life
5. Role play
6. Questionnaire

## Full Assessment (1–2 hours)

1. Interview
   - Where and when client speaks English
   - Any significant personal/professional problems related to accent
   - Questions about personal and professional life
   - Goals
2. Diagnostic passage (50–200 words)
   - "Please Call Stella," "Comma Gets a Cure," "Rainbow Passage," ACT diagnostic passage, etc.
3. Segmental assessment of all consonant and vowel phonemes
   - 15–30 words and sentences (see sample)
4. Listening discrimination with minimal pairs
5. Spontaneous speech sample
   - Speaking prompt
   - Picture description
6. Structured intonation assessment
7. Role play
8. Questionnaire
9. Grammar/vocabulary assessment
10. Writing sample
    - Use a writing prompt or have a client bring in samples

# 4

# Segmentals Overview

## Working with Sounds

Segmentals are the individual sounds of speech, and historically they have formed the basis of most accent modification work up until the last 30 to 40 years. The IPA, which is familiar to SLPs, came about as the result of language teachers working on a systematic way to teach sound systems to non-native speakers over one hundred years ago. While this book embraces a balance between segmentals and suprasegmentals to achieve the best results, the history of the field shows that the connection between a person's accent and the ability to produce the consonants and vowels of a language is self-evident. Segmentals are an area of strength for SLPs (especially in terms of the consonants) because of their training, depth of knowledge, and experience eliciting sounds.

## Phonemes and Allophones

A useful distinction that applies to segmentals is the difference between phonemes and allophones, and a quick review can help set the stage for working with speakers of other languages. A phoneme is a speech sound that can change the meaning of a word, and each language draws on its inventory of these phonemes to create its vocabulary. If we take the word *hat* and replace the initial /h/ with a /k/, we get *cat*, which is a fundamentally different entity. While typically-developing native speakers master these distinctions as toddlers, non-native speakers may never learn to accurately produce all of the sounds of their new language, and this can result in miscommunications. Non-natives can draw on their own inventories to produce sounds that are nearly identical to those in their L2, but if individual phonemes are missing from their L1 inventory, they may not be able to perceive them, or they may not be able to produce the necessary muscle movements to articulate them. Almost all non-native speakers of English who seek accent modification have had some formal English instruction, and since English is a widely taught foreign language, they generally have had some exposure in their school system before they arrive in an English-speaking country. When someone is learning a language, their teachers are bound to point out the phonemes of English that typically present challenges, so in most cases clients are aware of which sounds they have difficulty producing even though they may be uncertain about their exact nature. Since phonemes change meaning, non-native speakers are likely to discover quickly which ones are troublesome because native speakers will not understand a particular word they are trying to say. If a client says, "I'm waiting for the man to come," but produces *man* as /mɛn/, then a native will perceive this as plural and not singular; thus intelligibility is affected and the message is changed. Phonemes are therefore essential to successful communication and clients must master them in order to express themselves clearly.

Allophones are less powerful because they do not change the meaning of words. If we take the example of the word *hat* again, we can demonstrate how allophones work by producing the word first with a final released /t/, which will result in a clear, strongly enunciated version of the word. If we produce the word without an audible release of the final stop, as in [hæt̚], the production will probably sound more typical of the way it is pronounced in natural speech, but the meaning will not change. Non-native speakers may not be aware of these different options because the phonemes are said to be in free variation, meaning that speakers can choose freely between the two phonemes and neither one will not sound wrong. There is often a preference for one allophone or the other, depending on the formality of the situation, so clients need to increase their awareness of the options in order to fit in. Some allophones are essentially mandatory, as in the word *matter*, which speakers of American English produce as [mæɾɚ], with an alveolar tap and not a /t/. If non-native speakers produces the word with a /t/ then it will sound like [mætɚ], and the meaning is still the same. The difference here is that since native speakers of American English really never produce the word in this way, the non-native speaker will sound extremely unnatural. An important concept when working with both phonemes and allophones is that they are language specific, so something that is a phoneme in English might be an allophone in the client's language, and vice versa. There is one final idea related to allophones that can guide our work with clients. If a client says the word *hat* but produces it with a velar fricative /x/ (the sound sometimes used to say the *ch* in *loch* or *Bach*), native speakers are still likely to perceive it as *hat* and not *cat* because we do not use that sound as a phoneme in English, and they can recognize the speaker's intention. When non-native speakers substitute a sound not found in our language to produce a word that is still recognizable, we can think of it as a type of inappropriate allophonic variation. These types of substitutions will have less priority in accent modification work because they are less likely to disrupt communication, but in order to help clients sound more natural, these sounds should still be addressed.

Phonemic awareness is the ability to break down a word into its meaningful sounds. Since English has poor sound to symbol correspondence, our spelling system will generally be of little use in helping clients master pronunciation, so clinicians are better off using the IPA when we need to transcribe speech sounds. Although SLPs entering the world of accent modification might be rusty on their IPA transcription, they should have strong phonemic awareness, which is essential for anyone working with non-native clients. Clinicians must be able to take any word of English and describe exactly which phonemes are used to produce it. One objective of clinicians is to develop clients' phonemic awareness since it is extremely important for mastering the sound system of a language. While the IPA might come in handy during accent work for both the clinician and the client, phonemic awareness is the true goal, and the IPA is merely a tool to help develop it. After some training, clients should be able to break up English words into their constituent phonemes even if they never learn the phonetic symbols that represent them.

## International Phonetic Alphabet and Spelling

SLPs have a strong background in phonetics and phonology, and this is one reason they tend to have an advantage over TESOL instructors when it comes to providing accent modification services. When I trained ESL teachers in the Best Methods in Teaching Pronunciation and Fluency course at UCSD's English Language Institute, I spent a great deal of time teaching the IPA and developing teachers' phonemic awareness. Undergraduate courses in phonetics, which are required for ASHA certification, cover the IPA extensively and students develop good transcription skills that they later hone in graduate school. This book assumes that readers have a good grasp of both the problems associated with English orthography and the efficacy of the one-to-one sound to symbol correspondence of the IPA. Clients, on the other hand, may have only a limited awareness of this issue, and it is important to address it at an early stage of training. In most cases, clients need at most only a passive knowledge of some IPA symbols, but clients should learn to trust their ears and not their eyes when it comes to pronouncing English words.

The writing systems of the world's languages exist on a spectrum ranging from highly phonetic (e.g., Finnish, Korean, Ukrainian) to those such as Mandarin, that have very limited sound to symbol correspondence. Clients' attitudes toward English spelling are likely influenced by how it compares to their own in terms of transparency. During the early stages of training, it is often helpful to take spelling off the table by pointing out some of the extreme inconsistencies found in our system. The example of words ending in *ough* is a good way to illustrate this phenomenon. The words *cough*, *through*, *bough*, *thorough*, and *slough* are all pronounced with different endings despite their similar spellings. Clients need to know that there will be times when they can make judgments about the possible pronunciation of a word by the way it is written, and other times that it may as well be random. If clients ask why a word is spelled a certain way, it is usually helpful to point out that it simply does not matter when it comes to pronunciation, even if there is an interesting historical or etymological reason you can allude to.

When speakers learn their native language, they learn it by listening. Children of two or three years of age know how to say the word *cough* and what it means, but they are unlikely to be able to read it or spell it. When they learn to write, they begin by learning to match the words they already know how to produce to the way they are orthographically represented in our language. At a later stage this switches and children start to see words before they have heard them, but they quickly adapt to any mismatches between orthography and pronunciation. In contrast, most non-native speakers learn the sound of the word *cough* at the same time as they see its orthographic representation, which may result in some confusion. If non-native speakers learned the word *laboratory* /læbɹətɔɚi/ without ever seeing its spelling it is unlikely that they would ever produce it with an extra vowel between *lab* and *ratory*. The key is to shift our clients' focus away from these orthographic representations and encourage them to return to that childhood stage of language development where they relied entirely on sounds.

Although it is clear that the English spelling system is not reliable for identifying the pronunciation of all English words, there is still some degree of sound to symbol correspondence, so a case can be made for training clients to make educated guesses based on orthography. In Judy Gilbert's *Clear Speech* book (1997), she offers tips related to the frequency of symbols to sounds, for example, the letter *a* is pronounced as /æ/ 91% of the time. While this type of tip may offer some learners useful guidance, the chances are good that non-native speakers have already internalized many of the probable sound to symbol connections, and thus, should mainly focus on taking note of the exceptions. In the long run, clients are most likely to benefit from downplaying spelling and focusing on sounds as much as possible during accent training.

## Phonemic Awareness

Developing phonemic awareness (a term that can be made friendlier for clients by substituting *sound awareness*) is key to producing accurate segmentals. Clients do not need to learn any IPA symbols to be successful, but they should be able to take any English word and break it into phonemes, and using the IPA may help with that process. Once clients have been informed about difficulties of relying on spelling for pronunciation, they can focus on specific examples of spelling irregularities to clean up some possible spelling interference issues they may have and then stay on guard in the future. For example, the clinician can review words such as *salmon, cupboard, clothes,* and *say/said* and elicit the client's current pronunciation. If it strays from expectations, the differences between the written form and the pronunciation should be highlighted. Appendix 4–1 is a sample worksheet that can be used to focus on sound awareness and spelling irregularities.

The next stage in developing phonemic awareness might be to ask clients to identify which words in a set begin or end with the same consonant or feature the same vowel. For example, they could be asked to look at the words *use, young, unhappy, university* to find the odd man out to help develop awareness that the *u* letter sometimes represents a consonant (semivowel) and other times a vowel. If they identify the endings in a list such as *laughed, changed, slipped,* and *loved,* they should notice that only *slipped* ends in a /t/ sound, and this will help them focus on the rules for the pronunciation of regular past tense endings. Exercises identifying vowels should be especially effective since there is more variation in their pronunciation than for consonants. Another method to focus on sound instead of spelling is to show clients two words, and ask if the underlined or bolded letters in them represent the same sound. For example, if shown *f<u>oo</u>t* and *f<u>oo</u>d*, they should identify the words as having different vowel sounds, while the vowels in *s<u>ui</u>te* and *wh<u>ea</u>t* sound the same. Once clients are aware of the need to focus on sounds, work on specific difficult phonemes can come later in the training.

Introducing the concept of the IPA is a good way to reinforce the concepts above, and clinicians can decide on a case by case basis how much to rely on the IPA with their clients during training. Some clients will have become familiar with the IPA in their home countries, but for others, introducing it may present challenges that outweigh the benefits. Some accent books rely on a type of "eye dialect" spelling system to keep a closer connection to typical English spelling. For example, Ann Cook's *American Accent Training* book (Cook & Forsyth, 2017) uses a combination of English letters and special characters, especially to provide examples of connected speech, so "write it in a letter" comes out as "räididinə leddr." The IPA has the advantage of being well-developed and widely used, so it is still the first choice in accent work by far, but clinicians should always feel free to use any means necessary to bring about results. In some cases, clients with phonetic languages (especially those with larger phonemic inventories) simply use their own language to transcribe the way English words are actually pronounced, and clinicians have no reason to discourage this practice if it works. SLPs should also feel free to adjust the IPA to serve their purposes. In the same way that there is little need to use the /ɹ/ instead of /r/ when working with English alone, it is common to use the /y/ for the /j/ since English does not have the /y/ vowel, and our *j* letter is only pronounced as /j/ in loan words.

There is little benefit to training your clients extensively on the IPA, and there is really no reason for clients' knowledge not to be almost entirely passive. With regards to the vowels, it might make sense to show clients the entire quadrilateral with the IPA symbols just to give some definition to the vowel space, but there is certainly no need for them to memorize it. IPA symbols can be used sparingly to focus attention on a particular sound or sound contrast, and clinicians should be diligent about reminding clients of the sound the symbols represent by producing plenty of oral examples. Clinicians might also find that at times it can help to transcribe a word or short phrase and analyze it with the client while providing oral models. Appendix 4–2 lists the phonemes of English with keywords and can be given to clients as a reference guide.

The term *false friend* is used in linguistics to refer to words from two different languages that appear to be related but which have divergent meanings, for example the Spanish word *simpático* is related to the English word *sympathetic*, but whereas the Spanish word means nice or likable, the English word generally refers to showing compassion. A Spanish speaker acquiring English might say, "He's very sympathetic," when meaning "He's very nice," so a misunderstanding may result. There is a similar phenomenon which can happen with the pronunciation of words that look alike. Although these are not technically false friends, there is an analogous effect. To illustrate, the English word *natural* looks exactly like the Spanish word *natural*, and even though they have virtually identical meanings, the citation form of the English version is pronounced /næʧɚəl/ while the Spanish word is pronounced /natural/. A Spanish speaker is likely to do one or more of the following based on spelling and their familiarity with saying the word in their native language from an early age: substitute the /a/ for the /æ/, fail to reduce the other vowels, or substitute /t/ for /ʧ/. Note that the words do not have to be spelled exactly alike for this effect to occur, so the French word *naturel* may influence a non-native speaker to pronounce the English word *natural* with a /t/. Because English belongs to the Indo-European language family, which has the largest number of speakers in the world, coming in at twice that of the second place Sino-Tibetan family, many clients will speak languages related to English and clinicians may need to monitor for these kinds of mistakes. Although speakers of languages from other language families might make similar mistakes, they may actually benefit from having less to unlearn.

# Principles of Segmental Training

## Basic Techniques

SLPs come to the world of accent modification with a good grasp of methods for eliciting and shaping sounds, and our field has countless resources dedicated to this type of work. SLPs should apply all of their knowledge and experience when working to elicit and shape the sounds of non-native clients, and typically any adaptations that are required are relatively straightforward. The major difference with accent clients, compared to developmental work or work with speech-language disorders, is that accent clients do not typically have language disabilities or delays. The following are a few factors to keep in mind when working with accent modification clients. First of all, while they are typically highly motivated, they may not always complete assigned home practice, and it is important to motivate them in a respectful and encouraging way. In addition, they may have difficulties with comprehension, so clinicians must monitor their clients' level of understanding. SLPs working in accent modification need to develop good abilities to adapt their own vocabulary to clients' abilities in English. Generally, clients who seek accent modification services already have a high proficiency level, so it is less likely that they will be at a beginning or pre-intermediate level, but clinicians are still encouraged to focus on identifying which words cause them more difficulty. Clinicians who have experience working with children may benefit from past experience simplifying their own syntax and vocabulary. It is important not to appear to be talking down to clients since they are generally highly educated and neurotypical. On the other hand, clinicians may be tempted to use technical jargon or overly complex explanations since these clients have no cognitive impairments and are usually intelligent and successful, but this temptation should be avoided. The balance between excessive simplification and needless complexity must be based on each client's particular stage of second language acquisition, and while it is certainly a challenge to find that balance, it is something most SLPs working with non-native speakers learn to master. For SLPs who have learned a second language as an adult, it can be useful to reflect on which words and grammatical forms were acquired at various stages, and then use that awareness when speaking in English.

SLPs can use the same basic modeling and prompting techniques for accent modification that they use with children and adults who have communication disorders, and they

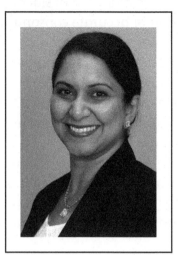

I think coming from a speech-language pathology background with knowledge of the articulatory and phonological systems and how to train individuals to modify their sound production is a large benefit. Also, while this is not therapy for a medically-related issue, having that practical experience of working and interacting with an individual through a training session utilizing a hierarchy of cueing, modifying stimulus materials, etc., is also quite beneficial in my corporate practice.

—Sonia Sethi Kohli, M.S, CCC-SLP The Global Speech Suite

can follow their instincts and training to determine the best ways to help clients acquire the segmentals. Since the clients are adults, they have a high tolerance for drills, but clinicians can use more imaginative activities to spice things up. For example, when working on particular sounds, clinicians can choose word lists that include items that are either of special interest to the client or are designed to expand their vocabularies. These strategies are key to providing meaningful practice. Idioms are also an excellent way to provide practice on selected segmentals while giving clients some exposure to another important element of natural sounding language use. Basically, everything is on the table during segmental training sessions; nonsense words, word lists, phrases, short paragraphs, picture descriptions, and tongue twisters, are just a few of the possible tools available. Clinicians can balance activities that involve controlled production of individual words focusing on a particular phoneme with activities that introduce opportunities to use spontaneous speech, and free-speaking activities that promote generalization. As an example of an activity from the middle range of the spectrum, clinicians can provide clients with nonsense sentences where the correction involves a target phoneme. For example, if the clinician is focusing on the *th* sound, the prompt can be something like "Thanksgiving is always on a Wednesday," and the client can correct it by saying, "Thanksgiving isn't on a Wednesday, it's always on a Thursday." The goal is for clients to practice producing sounds in a variety of contexts while the clinician provides feedback and modeling.

SLPs generally do not have much experience working with vowels, and there are a few things to keep in mind while working on these segmentals. Clinicians will certainly want to provide models of target vowel sounds and make an effort to explain some of the physiology involved. Describing the production of vowels can be challenging because there is no contact between articulators, so listeners must rely much more on their ears to shape their sounds. In some cases, jaw and lip position will be useful starting points to shape the client's efforts, but generally the clinician will shape productions through modeling and feedback, and clients will have to internalize the movements taking place out of sight and without the sensation of touch that might bolster their acquisition of accurate consonants. Basic drills can be effective, and since clients are adults, they have a higher tolerance for activities that children might find less engaging. These drills can include reading lists of words that contain the target vowel or repeating the clinician's models. A good case can be made for providing practice opportunities for target vowels in a variety of contexts, but certain contexts may be more useful than others at the beginning stages of training, when clients are developing confidence. Vowels in a stressed syllable are the most salient, and most clinicians tend to focus on one or two syllable words. Using consonant-vowel (CV) words for tense vowels or monosyllabic words that end in a final voiced consonant will take advantage of the allophonic rules for English vowel length. Clinicians can experiment with different contexts to determine which may be the most facilitative for accurate productions.

Visual feedback is certain to become an important tool as the technology that was once found only in research laboratories makes its way to handheld devices. Vowelviz (http://completespeech.com/vowelvizpro/) is low-cost software for Apple devices that allows clients to watch a cursor react to the vowels they produce and identify them on an IPA chart. The technology is not yet perfect, but it is certainly an indicator of what is to come. In addition, many clients use voice recognition software on their phones to monitor whether they are producing difficult vowels accurately.

Minimal pairs (see next section) are also valuable tools for helping clients master the vowels, and they can also be used diagnostically at an early stage in training to develop a better understanding of which contrasts are the most difficult for a client to distinguish or produce. They are particularly effective because clients may have greater difficulty perceiving the differences between vowels in comparison to many of the consonants. Clients can also work with sentences, whether natural sounding or improbable, that either contain many samples of the target vowel, such as, "Tim hit him with a whip," to focus on the /ɪ/ or with sentences that feature samples of both the target vowel and a partner vowel that is a typical substitution. An example of the latter type of sentence would be "Tim heats it with his team" to focus on the contrast between /i/ and /ɪ/. Clinicians can also use lengthy passages containing multiple samples of the target vowels, or even tongue twisters, to encourage generalization and awareness of phonemes.

## Minimal Pairs

Many SLPs receive their first exposure to minimal pairs in their undergraduate phonetics class when they learn about the concept of phonemes, and they often apply this knowledge at some point when working with children who have speech sound disorders. Minimal pairs are used extensively in accent modification because they are a highly effective way to identify and remedy phonemic inventory mismatches. There are occasional debates about their efficacy, and many researchers in the TESOL world decry their artificiality, but many clinicians swear by them, and clients generally have a fondness for them as well. One of my clients told me how much he loved the concept and praised minimal pairs for being scientific, and I concur with his assessment.

If you have not used minimal pairs for a while, the concept is simple. Minimal pairs are two words that differ in one sound only. That simple definition is all you need to know, but here are some additional details.

1. Spelling is irrelevant since we are only interested in sounds. For example, *go* and *dough* are minimal pairs, but *cow* and *tow* are not.

2. The two words in a minimal pair must have different meanings. Remember that sometimes we can change the way we say a sound in a word and we don't change the meaning. For example, we can release the final /t/ in "cat" or we can hold it, but that wouldn't change the meaning, so changing one sound does not always create a minimal pair.

3. Minimal pairs must also have the same number of sounds. Notice how the words *see/seed*, as shown in Table 4–1, are NOT a minimal pair. These are sometimes called *near minimals*, and they may also be effective tools when working on sounds. On the other hand, *tree* and *three* are minimal pairs. Table 4–2 shows how the number of phonemes is identical, and the substitution of /t/ for /θ/ produces a new word.

4. There has to be exactly one sound different, so *sun* and *son* are not minimal pairs because there is no sound that is different, and *food* and *foot*, as shown in Table 4–3, are not minimal pairs because two sounds are different.

5. The different sound can be in any position in the word, so all of the pairs in Table 4–4 are minimal pairs.

6. Words with just one phoneme can be minimal pairs, so *I* and *owe* are minimal pairs. There is no limit to the number of phonemes in a minimal pair, although they are harder to find the longer the words are, so most tend to be in the two to five phoneme range.

**Table 4–1.** Near Minimals

| s | i |   |
|---|---|---|
| s | i | d |

**Table 4–2.** Minimal Pair with /t, θ/ as the Only Difference

| t | r | i |
|---|---|---|
| θ | r | i |

**Table 4–3.** Pairs with Two Sound Differences Are Not Minimal Pairs

| f | u | d |
|---|---|---|
| f | ʊ | t |

**Table 4–4.** Minimal Pairs with Differences in Initial, Medial, and Final Phonemes

| b | u | t |
|---|---|---|
| s | u | t |

boot/suit

| b | ɪ | t |
|---|---|---|
| b | æ | t |

bit/bat

| b | ɝ | d |
|---|---|---|
| b | ɝ | n |

bird/burn

**Table 4–5.** Sample Minimal Pairs Chart

|   | A. "ch" /tʃ/ | B. "sh" /ʃ/ |
|---|---|---|
| 1 | chore | shore |
| 2 | watch | wash |
| 3 | switching | swishing |
| 4 | catch | cash |
| 5 | crutches | crushes |

The beauty of minimal pairs is that they allow us to isolate exactly which phoneme is causing a problem. If we are working with the minimal pairs *pin* and *bin* and the client tries to say *pin*, but it comes out as *bin*, then we know that the initial /p/ is a problem phoneme. Drilling with minimal pairs is a good way to focus the client on producing distinct sounds, and it provides data to demonstrate success. In the real world, minimal pairs can be a source of frustration for clients who have incomplete phonemic inventories for English; if a non-native speaker uses the /i/ vowel to produce *hit* it will come out as *heat*, which may result in a misunderstanding.

When working with minimal pairs, clients will generally be working with a chart, such as the one shown in Table 4–5. Numbering the rows of the chart allows you to easily direct clients to particular items. The columns are labeled with letters in case the actual sounds of the phonemes are difficult for clients to perceive or produce. Often, these tables are used for listening discrimination first in order to make sure that the client can hear the difference in the sounds, but it is important to note that evidence on the relationship between perception and production in accent modification is inconclusive. Derwing and Munro (2015, p. 36) point out that "poor production is not always tied to poor perception, and the reverse is also true." Another way to use the minimal pairs chart is for clinicians to simply choose a row, read out a word from one of the columns, and have the client respond with "A" or "B." As an introduction, it can be helpful to read through several (or all) of the columns so that clients can train their ear for the distinction, keeping in mind the caveat above. This chart is somewhat short, with only five rows of words, but often it is beneficial to have charts with 10–20 rows. At times, clinicians may want to use minimal sets to provide a larger range of targets, such as the sets shown in Table 4–6.

**Table 4–6.** Minimal Sets

|   | A. /æ/ | B. /ʌ/ | C. /ɑ/ |
|---|---|---|---|
| 1 | cab | cub | cob |
| 2 | bag | bug | bog |
| 3 | sack | suck | sock |

|   | A. /ɛ/ | B. /æ/ | C. /ʌ/ | D. /ɑ/ |
|---|---|---|---|---|
| 1 | den | Dan | done | Don |
| 2 | net | gnat | nut | knot |
| 3 | flex | flax | flux | flocks |

Again, to practice listening discrimination, clinicians can choose a single item and have clients identify the column, or they can read out two or more words. For example, in Table 4–6, clinicians can read out "done" and "Dan," and the client should say "C, B." Clinicians should always be ready to repeat items as needed. If a client is making good progress, the clinician might point to row 2 and say "nut, knot, nut" and the client can respond with "C, D, C." If clients are struggling with perception and feel that they are in a rut, clinicians can engage in production practice to see if gains can be made more rapidly that way. In any case in which a client begins to feel stuck, clinicians should work at finding a good way to push clients to achieve their potential without causing frustration.

Once clients have done well at the word level, a useful type of minimal pair activity is to use sentences like those in Table 4–7, which allow clients to work on the sounds in more natural contexts.

One other common technique is to have clients listen to choices and then respond accordingly, as shown in Table 4–8. This type of activity can be done with the prompts visible (as above) or hidden, in which case clients see only the possible choices and listen to the sentences spoken by the clinician, rather than read them.

**Table 4–7.** Minimal Pair Sentences

|   | A. /æ/ | B. /ʌ/ | C. /ɑ/ |
|---|---|---|---|
| 1 | The caps are there. | The cups are there. | The cops are there. |
| 2 | The cat is on the rug. | The cut is on the rug. | The cot is on the rug. |
| 3 | Did you see the bag? | Did you see the bug? | Did you see the bog? |

**Table 4–8.** Prompt and Response Minimal Pairs

|   | Prompt | Response |
|---|--------|----------|
| 1 | a.  The cops are here. | a.  Did someone break the law? |
|   | b.  The cups are here. | b.  Good. I'll pour a drink. |
| 2 | a.  Is that Don? | a.  Yes, I think that's him. |
|   | b.  Is that done? | b.  No. It's not quite finished. |

These are the most typical types of minimal pair activities, but clinicians can use their imagination to develop other engaging activities. Up to this point, all of the activities described have been for testing perception, but most of the time they are used to work on production. The principle is essentially the same, but now the clinician is the judge, and the client chooses which word to say. If a clinician listens to a word in isolation, it can be difficult to determine whether the segmentals were said with enough accuracy to avoid miscommunication, but using minimal pairs forces clinicians to choose between two possibilities, which makes it much easier to determine whether a client is able to produce the sounds distinctly. Clients enjoy minimal pairs, and they are an excellent way for both client and clinician to gauge progress.

## Other Auditory Discrimination Activities

Auditory discrimination activities establish whether a client can perceive differences in a pair or set of segmentals, and are especially useful when working with vowels. In contrast to methods often used with children, such as auditory bombardment, in which clients listen to target sounds without responding, in accent modification activities, clients are generally asked to respond to the stimulus. In addition to the use of minimal pairs, there are many other approaches that have been used to good effect. For example, clients can listen as a clinician reads pairs of words and then identify whether they feature the same or different vowels. If the clinician says, "bend/red," the client responds "same," and then for "send/stand," the client responds "different." Clients can also listen to words or short phrases and decide whether a particular phoneme is present or not, as in the following:

"Listen to the following words and tell me if a word has the /ɪ/ vowel, as in *hit*: beat, seat, lit, meet, pit, seep, leap, rip."

Another possibility is an "odd man out" activity, in which clients listen to four words and determine which one has (or does not have) a particular target phoneme, as in this example:

"Which word has the unvoiced 'th' as in *thin*: sink, zinc, think, fink?"

As mentioned above, the connection between perception and production is not clear from the research. Kartushina and Frauenfelder (2014, p. 2) provide an extensive review of studies and conclude, "the lack of converging results across different L2 perception-production studies could partially be due to the differences in the methods used (e.g., tasks, stimuli) and analyses applied (e.g., comparison of average performance in perception and production of a group of speakers versus correlation analysis across individuals). Nevertheless, taken together they point to the absence of a robust relationship between L2 perception and production." On an intuitive level, we can point to examples such as the trilled /r/ in Spanish, where English speakers have no difficulty identifying it perceptually, but often struggle to learn to produce it. There is some research indicating that hearing prompts from different voices and listening to phonemes with a wide range of allophonic variation is an effective way to promote the ability to discriminate sounds (Iverson, Hazan, & Bannister, 2005), but clinicians working one-on-one with clients may have difficulty putting this into practice. One option would be to use some recordings or videos as a supplement to their own productions. English Accent Coach (https://www.englishaccentcoach.com/) is a website that uses this approach. When working on phoneme discrimination, keep in mind that there is no need to wait until a client is completely successful at identifying the sounds before working on producing them; perception and production work can go hand in hand.

# Generalization

Generalization is often half (or perhaps more!) of the battle, and much of the work done with clients will involve promoting their ability to produce the segmentals in their everyday communication. This is a part of virtually everything SLPs do, and yet, it is also something that can be frustratingly elusive for clinicians and clients to achieve. And while both clinician and client are involved at the beginning, the whole point is for the client to take over in the end. There is no recipe book here—there are an infinite number of approaches and a staggering range of individual variation in our clients. As a starting point, clients need to know what is at stake when they are able to produce sounds in a controlled activity and not in everyday speech because this will help them focus on the goal more directly. Clinicians need to strike a balance between encouraging clients and pushing them hard when they struggle. Although this discussion focuses on segmentals, all of the techniques discussed can be adapted for suprasegmental targets as well.

---

I think the biggest challenge is when a client has to work against a long-established pattern of speech. I have clients who have spoken English with a strong accent for 30 years. It is difficult to help this kind of client make changes in his or her speech. Their patterns are strongly established. The errors have become fossilized. But it is not impossible! A client who practices can make changes and get the new pronunciation pattern to become automatic.

—Paula Gallay

Many clients face frustration when trying to apply what they have learned to their everyday speech. Sometimes, they feel that it will be impossible to produce sounds accurately without focusing on them. For example, when clients first learn that English universally lengthens vowels before final voiced consonants, they envision themselves analyzing each word carefully for several seconds before they utter it. There are several good analogies that might help build clients' confidence. For example, in sports and music, it is common to learn a new technique that requires a significant amount of attention at the beginning but becomes second nature with time. Clients can recall their experiences learning to drive a car; during their first driving lesson they probably need to concentrate carefully about starting the car, shifting gears, and applying the brakes, but when they drive now, they are probably barely conscious of their actions.

Although the list of activities to promote generalization is truly limitless, there are some ideas that can help clinicians get started as they discover approaches that work best. One effective avenue is to work with recordings. There are many possibilities here, but to start, tell the client that you are going to record for a minute or two and monitor for a particular sound. For example, for a French speaker, it might be /h/. You can use your phone, your client's phone, or both. An advantage to using the client's phone is that they will have a record of the activity. The actual speaking task can be anything, such as a basic conversation starter (e.g., "What did you do last night?" "Tell me about your best friend.") to a fun "Would you rather . . . ?" type question. Once a minute or two have passed, you can listen to the recording together. It is a good idea to try different techniques here. Often, at the beginning, clinicians can point out all of the accurate and inaccurate productions of a target phoneme, but later, it is highly recommended that clients take over and judge each production. Clients can designate errors by raising their hand, calling out the word, or taking notes, and the clinician can give feedback. One option is for both the clinician and client to make notes and then compare judgments. Both can tally accurate (or inaccurate) productions and compare totals. Once the client has had some experience with this, there are some helpful extensions of the activity. The recording can be longer, with all or only a portion reviewed later, or clinicians can record much longer chunks of the session, and then randomly stop to review the tape with the client. Clinicians can also set up the activity as above without identifying which target will be reviewed. If clients are working on several segmental goals, they will need to monitor several things at once.

Many engaging production tasks can be done without recording, and as above, clients can be told what to monitor or not. With these activities, the clinician can decide how to review target productions. One possibility is to "catch" clients with an inaccurate production by raising a hand or making a tally mark, and another option might be to simply review the productions impressionistically and possibly cite an example. Speaking tasks that work well for this are boundless, and might include picture descriptions, provocative questions, role plays, and story retells, to name a few. Clinicians can also work with clients to develop signals for specific sounds and then use them intermittently to indicate that the sound was produced accurately.

Another useful method to promote generalization is distraction. One method to distract is for clinicians to interject a question or comment during a more structured activity.

For example, while a client is focused on the accurate production of a specific sound during an activity, the clinician can say something like, "Oh, I forgot to ask you about . . ." and then change the subject to see if carryover occurs. An accomplice can also enter the room and engage with the client.

The late Pam Marshalla's wonderful book *Carryover Techniques in Articulation and Phonological Therapy* (2010) is an excellent resource containing feedback ideas collected from dozens of practicing SLPs, and one of the many ideas is the use of key words, which are words containing a target sound for clients to conscientiously produce with extra attention. For example, a Spanish-speaking client who is working on voicing fricatives might use the word *easy* as a key word and pay special attention to producing a /z/ in that word on every occasion.

Clinicians should view every interaction with their client at the beginning of a new session as an opportunity to measure progress since clients are usually less likely to monitor during the initial small talk. And since the ultimate goal is to have clients produce target sounds outside of sessions, to promote generalization clients can make a phone call, or go outside and find a real person to talk to. Clients can also be encouraged to try several things at home. They can record themselves in conversation (with their interlocutor's permission, of course), or they can keep a diary and jot down a few notes every day with a subjective review of how well they produced targets during their conversations.

---

Many clients can make progress within a treatment session. The challenge is finding the best way to motivate clients to *continue* practicing outside of the session (this is always the challenge in every setting)!

—Julie Cunningham

---

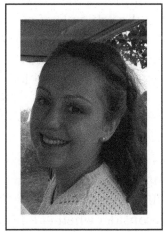

The program helped me gain knowledge of how to pronounce English words and sounds correctly, and now I can feel that it has generalized to almost all of the words I use. Now I feel that I do not have to make extra effort to sound more natural and it makes me feel more competent, and hence, more confident at my job when communicating orally with native English speakers. In addition, people stopped asking me twice about what I want at drive-through places! I think it is okay to have an accent, especially when it is not so noticeable.

—Irina Shubina, Accent Modification Client

# Target Selection

In most cases, clients need to work on a variety of segmental and suprasegmentals to improve their intelligibility and naturalness, and it is important to select targets carefully to maximize efficiency. There are several methods for determining which segmentals should be targeted, and good clinicians will review a number of factors to make this determination. In the TESOL world, when conducting a course designed for a group of multilingual, non-native speakers, targets can be selected in advance by identifying which English segmentals tend to be most challenging for the largest number of students, but this approach would not be efficient for SLPs working with individual clients or small groups. A good segmental assessment and a thoughtful analysis of the most important targets using the principles outlined below will help SLPs develop an efficient training program.

## Contrastive Analysis

Robert Lado laid the groundwork for the use of contrastive analysis in his book *Linguistics Across Cultures* in 1957, and during the 1960s and 1970s his approach was popular in the field of second language acquisition. Its application to target selection in accent modification involves comparing the phonemic inventory of a client's L1 with the phonemic inventory of English. If a phoneme is present in English and not in the client's L1, then it becomes a suitable target. For example, Spanish lacks the /z/ phoneme, and thus, it would be targeted. In addition, phonotactics are taken into account. Russian fully devoices final voiced consonants, so accent modification with Russian-speaking clients should focus, in part, on increasing the voicing in that context. Allophones are also considered, so if a client speaks a language that produces unvoiced initial stops with less aspiration than English, this could be targeted as well. Contrastive analysis will almost always be used to some extent to determine which targets are most suitable for accent modification because segmental contrasts between languages are what create problems with intelligibility and naturalness. SLPs who build up experience working with clients from one linguistic background will develop a good understanding of the phonemic inventories of their clients' L1 and become adept at listening for these differences. To highlight the principle of contrastive analysis, we can compare the phonemic inventories of South American Spanish with English to determine some potential targets. Clinicians can find phonemic inventories in resources such as the *Handbook of the IPA*, or find the information online. If we look at the consonant inventories of South American Spanish and English, we can create a chart that shows which phonemes are unique to each language and which are found in both languages, as illustrated in Table 4–9.

We can then focus on the subset of English only consonants because we would expect Spanish-speaking clients to have difficulty with them. As mentioned above, it is important to consider allophonic variations, so we may still find differences in the way the shared consonant phonemes are produced. We will also need to consider whether different dialects of South American Spanish feature different sets of phonemes. For example, the

**Table 4–9.** Contrastive Analysis South American Spanish and English Consonants

| Spanish only Consonant Phonemes | Shared Consonant Phonemes | English only Consonant Phonemes |
|---|---|---|
| /x, r, ɲ, ɾ / | /b,d,g,p,t,k,m,n,s,j,l,f,tʃ/ | /ʤ,v,ʃ,ʒ,ɹ,ŋ,θ,ð,z/ |

**Table 4–10.** Contrastive Analysis English and Spanish Vowels

| Spanish only Vowel Phonemes | Shared Vowel Phonemes | English only Vowel Phonemes |
|---|---|---|
| /a,o,e/ | /i,u/ | /ɪ,ɛ,æ,ɑ,ə,ʌ,ʊ,eɪ,oʊ,aɪ,aʊ,ɔɪ/ |

phonemic inventory of Spanish spoken in Spain features the /θ/ as a phoneme, while the Spanish dialects of South America do not. While English dialects differ primarily in terms of vowels, there is much more variation in the consonant inventories of the various dialects of Spanish, and it is important to be mindful of these differences when comparing inventories. Table 4–10 compares the vowel inventories of the two languages. Despite the fact that many of the differences in vowel phonemes are minor (e.g., Spanish has the monophthong /e/, but not the diphthong /eɪ/), we can see that Spanish lacks most of the vowels found in the English sound system.

Contrastive analysis does not indicate a client's abilities to produce segmentals accurately, it merely highlights differences in phonemic inventories, so it is always important to use it as a framework for expectations and not an indication of current levels. While it is certainly an efficient means to focus attention on the most likely segmental issues a client will have, there is a wide range of individual variation. Identifying inaccurate or absent segmentals in the target language is only one part of the target selection process. SLPs can increase the effectiveness of their work by prioritizing segmentals using a number of other principles, which are outlined below. As with contrastive analysis, when using other models to predict which sounds might be the most difficult for non-natives to acquire, such as Best's perceptual assimilation model (Best, McRoberts, & Sithole, 1988) or Flege's speech learning model (1995), clinicians must focus on the phonemes and allophones actually produced inaccurately by the client, regardless of whether they fit a particular model or not. SLPs are advised to heed Derwing and Munro's (2015, p. 75) advice that "error prediction is of limited value as a pedagogical resource and may actually lead to a misplaced focus . . ."

## Functional Load

A theoretical approach that has gained traction in recent years is the idea of choosing segmental targets based on their functional load. Functional load refers to the relative power of a phonemic contrast in a particular language. In each language, phonemes are used to create the sound distinctions that drive meaning, and in theory, some of these contrasts play a much greater role than others. Therefore, a contrast with a higher functional load would represent a more valuable target when working on second language phonology because it would have the greatest impact on intelligibility. The two pioneers of the application of this approach to pronunciation training are Catford (1987) and Brown (1991), who each created systems to analyze the relative importance of particular phonemic contrasts. The two models are somewhat complicated, but relatively similar, and are based on factors such as how many minimal pairs exist for each vowel pair, how common the words are in those pairs, and whether the words are of the same lexical class. In addition, a phoneme may be considered to have a lower functional load if it is not present in all dialects of the language. The phonemes /i, ɪ/ are said to have a high functional load since there are literally hundreds of minimal pairs based on these vowels, including many with high frequency words of the same lexical class. Native speakers who have no experience working with accents are generally aware of the problems associated with speakers who are unable to produce the lax vowel /ɪ/ and may be misunderstood when they say what sounds like "I leave here" when they mean "I live here." This contrast has a high functional load because it is easy to rattle off lists of minimal pairs such as beat/bit, heat/hit, tin/teen without much effort. In contrast, the vowels /u, ʊ/ would have a low functional load because there are very few minimal pairs, these pairs feature low frequency words, and the pairs feature words representing different parts of speech. It takes some effort to think of minimal pairs for /u, ʊ/, and those that come to mind, such as cooed/could, Luke/look feature low-frequency words from different lexical classes, and it is unlikely they would cause any misunderstanding. Some studies (Munro & Derwing, 2006 and Levis & Cortes, 2008) have shown a correlation between errors involving high functional load and miscommunications and between lower accentedness and comprehensibility ratings.

The advantages of a functional load approach is that clinicians can use a systematic analysis to determine a hierarchy of targets if they are focusing on intelligibility. Clinicians may be tempted to focus on a target such as /ʒ/ if the client is unable to produce it, but by analyzing functional load, another target which may have a greater impact on intelligibility would take precedence. This approach is a major reason that many researchers of pronunciation have argued against work on the interdentals /θ, ð/ even though they are two of the most common phonemes addressed in pronunciation textbooks and targeted in sessions.

There are also several reasons why this approach may not be ideal. First, functional load rankings are based on theoretical criteria that have not been fully tested. There is no universally agreed upon method to determine functional load, and there is only limited evidence demonstrating a clear connection between these rankings and the appropriateness of particular segmental targets. While some research has sought to demonstrate that typical targets addressed in materials designed for pronunciation work are not related to functional load principles, from a practical point of view, a more likely concern might be how disconnected these rankings are from the typical work carried out by those working in accent modification. As an example, Table 4–11 lists the top six consonant contrasts identified by Catford (1987) and Brown (1988) as having the highest functional load.

**Table 4–11.** High Functional Load Consonant Phoneme Pair Rankings

| Ranking | Catford Initial Consonants | Brown |
|---------|---------------------------|-------|
| 1 | /k,h/ | /p,b/ |
| 2 | /p,b/ | /p,f/ |
| 3 | /p,k/ | /m,n/ |
| 4 | /p,t/ | /n,l/ |
| 5 | /p,h/ /s,h/ | /l,ɹ/ |
| 6 | /l,ɹ/ | /f,h/ |

Of the items on this list, only /l,ɹ/ are common target pairs in accent modification, and are especially common for clients from Japan. In addition, /p,f/ is targeted when working with several languages (including Korean), /p,b/ may be targeted when working with clients who speak Arabic, and /n,l/ are sometimes targets for speakers of some dialects of Mandarin Chinese, but apart from those pairs, the other target pairs are extremely rare if not entirely nonexistent as targets. It is easy to see why /p,t/ are considered to have a high functional load because there are so many minimal pairs featuring this contrast, and many of those pairs feature words of the same lexical class. Nevertheless, these two sounds are extremely common in the world's languages, and it is highly unlikely that a client would not be able to produce distinct versions of these phonemes. If we isolate the individual phonemes from these pairs, we have /p,t,k,b,m,n,f,s,h,ɹ,l/, and of this list, only /ɹ/ stands out as an extremely common target. Other phonemes such as /h,f,l/ are indeed targeted for speakers of several languages that are commonly spoken by clients in the United States, but in general they are not high on the list of the targets typically addressed in accent modification in this country.

If we approach this from the other direction, we can identify pairs considered to have low functional load that are valuable targets when working with non-native clients. Table 4–12 shows a list of selected items from both Catford's and Brown's analyses that are considered to have low functional load. These are not the last items on either author's list, but rather, they were chosen from the lower portion of their rankings to demonstrate that many typical targets are low on the list. These are all common segmental pairs that are addressed during training sessions.

Accent modification with a Spanish speaker is likely to focus on /ʃ,tʃ//d,ð//θ,t/ /dʒ,j//tʃ,dʒ//s,z/, for example, and that would represent a great number of the pairs in Table 14–12. Work with speakers of many other languages would also involve some or most of these contrasts. If we line up these phonemes individually, we get /t,d,f,v,θ,ð,s,z,ʃ,j,tʃ,dʒ,w/, and of this list /f,v,θ,ð,tʃ,dʒ,w/ are all fairly common targets in accent reduction. Thus, if we compare the consonant phonemes assigned higher rankings with those assigned lower rankings there is not a strong connection between hypothetical functional load and popularity as an accent modification target.

**Table 4–12.** Low Functional Load Consonant Phoneme Pair Rankings

| Ranking out of 48 | Catford | Ranking out of 28 | Brown |
|---|---|---|---|
| 32/48 | /ʃ,tʃ/ | 19/28 | /d,ð/ |
| 33/48 | /v,w/ | 22/28 | /θ,t/ |
| 35/48 | /dʒ,j/ | 23/28 | /tʃ,dʒ/ |
| 37/48 | /t,θ/ | 24/28 | /ʃ,tʃ/ |
| 44/48 | /s,z/ | 27/28 | /f,θ/ |
| 48/48 | /θ,ð/ /ð,z/ | 28/28 | /dʒ,j/ |

**Table 4–13.** High Functional Load Vowel Phoneme Pair Rankings

| Ranking | Catford Vowels | Brown Vowels |
|---|---|---|
| 1 | /ɪ,æ/ | /e*, æ/ |
| 2 | /i,ɪ/ | /æ ,ʌ/ |
| 3 | /ɔ,oʊ/ | /æ,ɒ/ |
| 4 | /ɪ,eɪ/ | /ʌ,ɒ/ |
| 5 | /æ,ɑ/ | /ɔː, əʊ/ |
| 6 | /æ,ʌ/ | /e*, ɪ/ |

*This would usually be transcribed as /ɛ/.

Table 4–13 outlines Catford's and Brown's top vowel phoneme contrasts. Of this collection, the /i,ɪ/ pair is the most typical segmental target, and in this case, Catford's ranking of second place lines up well with common practice. Incidentally, Brown ranks it at tenth out of 26. In accent modification, /ɛ, æ/ is a common target, and many languages do not feature either vowel. In addition, if we substitute /ɑ/ for /ɒ/ since American English does not use the latter phoneme, we find another common pair: /ʌ, ɑ/. The other pairs listed in the table are not common targets, but in contrast to the rankings of the consonant, the individual phonemes are indeed typically addressed in accent reduction work. If we isolate the vowel phonemes from their pairs, /ɪ,æ,ʌ,ɛ/ are all common segmental targets.

If we select vowel phoneme pairs that are ranked low on Catford's list, we have: /oʊ,aʊ/,/ɑ,ɔ/, /ɑ,ʊ/,/ʊ,ʌ/,/aɪ,aʊ/ "pin"/"pen." It's more difficult to analyze Brown's lower ranking vowels since his order reflects the Received Pronunciation dialect of British English and not American English. Catford's low-ranking vowels appear to line up better with typical accent modification practice since they are not typically addressed. In fact, /ɑ,ɔ/ would not typically be distinguished by the large number of American English speakers who have merged these vowels themselves.

In conclusion, the principle of functional load may be useful in selecting or ranking targets that are most likely to affect intelligibility. Vowel pairs such as /i,ɪ/ (ranked 2nd by

Catford, and 10th by Brown) are commonly contrasted in our language and are much more likely to lead to misunderstandings than vowel phonemes such as /u,ʊ/, which are featured in only a few rare minimal pairs. On the other hand, there is no universally agreed upon ranking of functional load, and it would be impractical to adhere rigorously to any that have been proposed. Clinicians should use their judgment when applying these principles and will perhaps find the most success when blending these ideas with other important considerations.

## Other Factors in Target Selection

The principle of functional load is most clearly connected to intelligibility, but in many cases clinicians may need to consider naturalness as well. A case in point would be the /t, θ/ contrast, which is ranked relatively low on the functional load rankings discussed above. It is actually very common for clients to substitute either a /t/ or an /s/ for the /θ/ since it is absent in the phonemic inventories of most of our clients. Listeners will adapt to this type of substitution, but they will make note of it, and even though intelligibility will not be significantly reduced, there will be an impact on the naturalness of speech. At other times, a client may produce an inappropriate allophonic variation. For example, a client from India might use a retroflex /t/, and there will be no doubt about the intended phoneme, but it will sound significantly different and native speakers will focus on how the client is speaking as opposed to what is being said. Intelligibility should always take precedence over naturalness, but SLPs need to be careful to monitor differences that can play a role in how non-native speech is perceived, as opposed to simply how it is understood.

Clinicians can base some of their targeting on stimulability and ease. During the assessment process, it may become clear that particular phonemes are within a client's immediate reach while others are more elusive. Often, clinicians can rack up some early victories by cleaning up these easier targets first, but in other cases, these targets can wait if they have less impact on intelligibility and the clinician feels that other targets need immediate attention. Psychologically, clients can benefit from the increased motivation that can come from acquiring a sound (or even awareness of sound differences) rapidly. Clinicians also have to balance segmental priorities with the client's suprasegmental needs, and those aspects of speech will be analyzed in detail in chapters to come.

## References

Best, C. T., McRoberts, G. W., & Sithole, N. M. (1988). Examination of perceptual reorganization for nonnative speech contrasts: Zulu click discrimination by English speaking adults and infants. *Journal of Experimental Psychology: Human Perception and Performance, 14*(3), 345–360.

Brown, A. (1988). *TESOL Quarterly, 22* (4), 593–606.

Brown, A., (1991). Functional load and the teaching of pronunciation. In Brown, A. (Ed.), *Teaching English pronunciation: A book of readings* (pp. 221–224). London, UK: Routledge.

Carney, E. (2014). *Survey of English spelling*. London, UK: Routledge.

Catford, J. C. (1987). Phonetics and the teaching of pronunciation: A systemic description of English phonology. In J. Morley (Ed.), *Current perspectives on pronunciation: Practices anchored in theory* (pp. 87–100). Washington, DC: TESOL.

Cook, A., & Forsyth, H. (2017). *American accent training: A guide to speaking and pronouncing colloquial American English*. Hauppauge, NY: Barrons.

Derwing, T. M., & Munro, M. J. (2015). *Pronunciation Fundamentals: Evidence-based perspectives for L2 teaching and research*. Philadelphia, PA: John Benjamins Publishing Company.

Flege, J. E. (1995). Second-language speech learning: Theory, findings, and problems. In W. Strange (Ed.), *Speech perception and linguistic experience: Theoretical and methodological issues* (pp. 233–277). Timonium, MD : York Press.

Gilbert, J. B. (2017). *Clear speech from the start: Basic pronunciation and listening comprehension in North American English*. Cambridge, UK: Cambridge University Press

Iverson, P., Hazan, V., & Bannister, K. (2005). Phonetic training with acoustic cue manipulations: A comparison of methods for teaching English /r/-/l/ to Japanese adults. *Journal of the Acoustical Society of America, 118*(5), 3267–3278.

Kartushina, N., & Frauenfelder, U. H. (2014). On the effects of L2 perception and of individual differences in L1 production on L2 pronunciation. *Frontiers in Psychology, 5*, 1–17.

Lado, R. (1957). *Linguistics across cultures*. Ann Arbor, Michigan: University of Michigan Press.

Levis, J., & Cortes, V. (2008). Minimal pairs in spoken corpora: Implications for pronunciation assessment and teaching. In C. A. Chapelle, Y. R. Chung, & J. Xu (Eds.), *Towards adaptive CALL: Natural language processing for diagnostic language assessment* (pp. 197–208). Ames, IA: Iowa State University.

Marshalla, P. (2010). *Carryover techniques in articulation and phonological therapy*. Kirkland, WA: Marshalla Speech and Language.

Munro, M., & Derwing, T. (2006). The functional load principle in ESL pronunciation instruction: An exploratory study. *System, 34* 520–531.

# 4-1

# English Spelling

1. Look at the following words. How do we pronounce them in English? How do you think the spelling might cause problems with pronunciation?

| | | | |
|---|---|---|---|
| sword | salmon | debt | says |
| choir | numb | heir | cupboard |

2. Sound Awareness

A.   Word Beginnings: Do the following words **start** with the same sound?

| Words | Same Sound | Different Sound |
|---|---|---|
| **ch**ef, **s**ugar | ✓ | |
| **u**niverse, **un**lucky | | |
| **kn**ight, **pn**eumonia | | |
| **j**eans, **g**eriatric | | |
| **th**in, **th**em | | |
| **ph**ase, **f**ace | | |
| **Ch**icago, **ch**ance | | |

B.   Word Endings: Do the following words **end** with the same sound?

| Words | Same Sound | Different Sound |
|---|---|---|
| te**ch**, ri**ch** | | ✓ |
| talke**d**, judge**d** | | |
| ba**th**, ba**the** | | |

| | | |
|---|---|---|
| buzz, surprise | | |
| cats, dogs | | |
| wish, which | | |
| massage, message | | |

C.    Word Middles: Do the following words have the same sound in the **middle**?

| Words | Same Sound | Different Sound |
|---|---|---|
| heat, hit | | ✓ |
| pleasure, pleasant | | |
| wand, band | | |
| gun, gone | | |
| said, plaid | | |
| foot, food | | |
| easy, greasy | | |

# English Speech Sounds

**Consonants**

/p/ pie
/t/ tie
/k/ cat
/b/ baby
/d/ dog
/g/ guy
/w/ want
/j/ yes
/l/ light
/r/ right
/m/ might
/n/ night
/ŋ/ ring
/f/ few
/v/ view
/s/ see
/z/ zoo
/θ/ thanks
/ð/ this
/h/ hot
/ʃ/ shoe
/ʒ/ beige, pleasure
/tʃ/ church
/dʒ/ judge

## Vowels

/i/ heat
/ɪ/ hit
/ɛ/ bed
/æ/ hat
/ɑ/ father
/ɔ/ for
/ʊ/ good
/u/ too
/ʌ/ bug
/ɝ/ word

## Unstressed Vowels

/ə/ potato
/ɚ/ farmer

## Diphthongs (double vowels)

/eɪ/ hate
/oʊ/ go
/aɪ/ lie
/aʊ/ out
/ɔɪ/ boy

CHAPTER

# 5

# Suprasegmentals
# Overview

## Patterns of Speech

The term *suprasegmentals* refers to any elements of speech beyond the level of individual sounds. The binary division of speech into segmental and suprasegmental levels may be somewhat artificial since they are always intertwined in communication, but this distinction is a useful construct that helps clinicians and clients focus on important aspects of pronunciation. Just as clients will benefit from an awareness of how spoken English works at the suprasegmental level, SLPs should take some time to develop their own understanding of these features in order to help their clients make gains. This chapter gives an overview of the major aspects of speech at the suprasegmental level and addresses two important features that should be emphasized early in training: intonation and rate.

Training on suprasegmentals is one of the most effective ways to help non-native clients become more effective communicators. SLPs are experts at communication, but they often need to develop their own awareness of suprasegmentals when they enter the field of accent modification. There are two main reasons for this. First, SLPs tend to have less experience providing therapy on suprasegmentals since most of their work with native speaking clients involves the accurate production of segmentals, and second, if they themselves are native speakers, they may have little explicit understanding of factors involved in producing natural sounding English speech. SLPs are generally most comfortable when eliciting segmentals and they may be less likely to concentrate on suprasegmentals. In the world of TESOL, awareness of the importance of suprasegmentals came relatively late. While some pioneers began to promote the importance of suprasegmentals (especially intonation) in L2 phonological acquisition shortly after World War II, it was not until the 1970s and 1980s that pedagogical theory began to affect practice. A survey of older training materials designed for non-native speakers reveals that they focused almost entirely on segmentals, and even today, many books aimed at self-study for accent modification are dedicated only to segmentals. While in some cases, particular clients may need significantly more work on the individual sounds of a language as opposed to the patterns that come into play in connected speech, in general, most clients need to address both levels in order to achieve maximal outcomes.

Clinicians should invest some time outlining the differences between the two levels for clients since this will help them analyze their own speech and prioritize goals. Clients often have some understanding of suprasegmental features, but it is rare for them to list any when asked about the challenges they face with English. Clients are quick to report that they have difficulty with the *r* or *th* and almost never mention intonation, phrasing, or rate. When referring to segmentals and suprasegmentals, it helps to simply call them "sounds" and "patterns" since the official terminology may be intimidating. At an early stage in accent training, clinicians can discuss these concepts and provide some examples. I often use the analogy of a house, in which the segmentals are individual bricks that are uniform and carefully crafted, and the suprasegmentals are the architecture. Providing clients with some typical examples of issues that non-native speakers have at segmental and suprasegmental levels allows clients to begin analyzing their own speech in those terms. The following are some examples of awareness building exercises:

1. Toshi has real problems hearing the difference between /r/ and /l/. The words "right" and "light" sound the same to him.

2. Chen does not connect words when he speaks, so many Americans tell him that his speech sounds choppy.

Clients can discuss these scenarios and decide if the problem is segmental or suprasegmental. Appendix 5–1 is a sample worksheet for developing awareness. Once clients have worked on this concept, ask them for examples of challenges they face on each level. Although segmental challenges may come to mind more readily, identifying suprasegmentals with precision often requires more instruction.

Just as it is helpful to provide clients with an overview of the consonants and vowels of English before working on them, clients can benefit from a tour of the suprasegmentals. Since most clients who seek accent modification have high-intermediate to advanced proficiency English, they should be ready to tackle any of the suprasegmentals, but in my experience, rate and intonation are often the first choices for clients of any proficiency level because those features have the greatest global impact.

# Rate

## Should Clients Slow Down?

Although other aspects of suprasegmentals are addressed in an introductory fashion in this chapter, and will be examined in more detail later in the book, the topic of speech rate is investigated in detail only in this chapter. Many SLPs target rate when helping clients with various communicative disorders, such as fluency, dysarthria, and autism spectrum disorder, and as a result of their training, SLPs are, to some extent, constantly monitoring the speed of the speech stream that surrounds them in their professional and personal lives. In the world of accent modification, there is a tendency to focus on slowing clients' speech in an effort to improve their intelligibility, but this book will make the case that in most circumstances, clinicians should actually aim to increase speech rate. By doing so, they will most likely increase naturalness of their clients' speech. Also, and perhaps counterintuitively, research suggests that increasing speech rate also boosts intelligibility. It is important to note that clinicians should always consider slowed rate of speech as one of many effective strategies in their arsenal to increase accuracy during accent modification, but the end goal for spontaneous speech should be a natural rate, and this generally means that the client should focus on speaking somewhat faster.

During a panel presentation on accent modification at a recent ASHA convention I attended, the suggestion that non-native speakers might benefit by increasing their rates was met with skepticism by many practitioners in the audience, so it is important to step back to analyze why conventional wisdom suggests a slower speech approach. This is most likely due to a general bias that SLPs have for intelligibility over naturalness, as discussed in previous chapters. When working with children's phonological delays it is advantageous to focus on slow and accurate articulation because the child's connected speech rate will never need to be the focus of attention. If intelligibility is compromised by a speech sound disorder, slower speech will most likely improve comprehensibility and once the child's delay has been remediated, the rate of speech will regress to the mean. In addition, slowing a dysfluent client's rate of speech has a long tradition in the field, so many clinicians may have had some experience using this approach in graduate school or in their practices. Unfortunately, when working with our accent clients, this advice may make them sound less natural and even reduce their intelligibility.

In a groundbreaking study, Munro and Derwing (1998) looked at which rates native speakers prefer when listening to non-native speakers and found that the listeners actually rated speech produced at a faster rate as more intelligible and less accented. They carried out a follow-up study in 2001 and found a similar result, and to date there has been no evidence to contradict their findings. Non-native speech that was either produced at a slower rate or digitally slowed down worsened listener ratings, and speech which was sped up digitally scored higher. Overall, they found that native speakers preferred rates that are slower than typical native speaker rates but faster than average non-native rates. As a side note, the notion that slowed speech reduces intelligibility goes back to at least 1943, when Fries, who collaborated with the pioneer in the study of intonation Kenneth Pike, stated that "slow speech hinders the comprehension of normal English" (Fries, 1943, p. 102). As with all research, results should be examined carefully to determine applicability, but clinicians should keep these findings in mind when attempting to balance the intelligibility and naturalness of their clients' speech.

When we ask clients whether natives or non-natives generally speak English faster, they virtually always answer that natives speak faster, and evidence supports their intuition (Derwing, Rossiter, Munro, & Thomson, 2004). There may be some cases where non-natives seem to speak English faster than natives (and in my experience these speakers tend to be from India or East Africa), but this may actually be more related to phrasing and stress issues, which can create the illusion of faster than average speech. For the most part, it is safe to say that clients seeking accent modification will not speak English faster than natives, so clinicians who are asking them to do so are clearly doing it to boost intelligibility and not naturalness.

Some clients will argue that they are speaking English slowly either because speech is generally slower in their language or because they happen to be slow speakers in their L1. There is some evidence that speech rate may be faster in various languages, with Germanic languages such as English reportedly slower than Romance languages (Polyanskaya, Ordin, & Busa, 2017), just as there is evidence that the norms may be different in some dialects of English (Jacewicz, Fox, O'Neill, & Salmons, 2009), but the overall difference between native and non-native should still play a larger role. Anderson-Hsieh and Venkatagiri (1994) reported that the mean articulation rate (syllables minus pauses) for native speakers of English was 5, while for highly proficient L2 English speakers it was 4.4 and for intermediate speakers it was 3.3. A study of air traffic controllers who had to pass an English oral proficiency test in order to work in their profession (Cauldwell, 2007) showed a correlation between levels achieved on the test and rate. Students who achieved level 3 (which was below passing) averaged 100 words per minute, while level 4 (passing) averaged 130 words per minute and level 5 (highest) averaged 180 words per minute. There is also evidence that speakers are slower in their L2 regardless of their idiolectic L1 rate. Hincks (2010) looked at speakers who spoke Swedish as a mother tongue and had high proficiency in their L2 English and compared identical presentations they gave in each language. Her findings showed that the non-natives were on average 23% slower when speaking, and that all of the speakers were slower in English than in their L1.

In the final analysis, we should expect our clients to speak English slower than natives, and slower than they speak their own language. It will always be important to use clinical judgment to determine what an appropriate rate is for each client. Just as pushing clients to speak faster than their abilities or at a rate that sounds unnatural is likely to have an impact on their communicative effectiveness, so will having them speak significantly slower than natives. The evidence from Munro and Derwing is clear—for most of our clients, encouraging them to speak faster than they currently do, but slower than natives, will generally result in more effective communication, and this approach fits well with an accent modification approach focusing on clear and natural speech.

## Measuring Rate

Speech rate has been studied from many angles, and the results have not always been consistent. One of the biggest challenges has been to determine which method of measuring will yield the most important information. Some of the most common methods focus on words per minute, syllables per minute (or per second), or articulatory rate, which refers to the rate of speech production minus pauses. Words per minute is probably the easiest to count, and it can be argued that it is an efficient way to ballpark how quickly someone can convey a message. Articulatory rate, on the other hand, would probably be too time consuming for our purposes, and it also has the disadvantage of eliminating all pauses, including appropriate pauses that may be the key to our clients' naturalness. Goetz (2013) points to studies showing that articulation rate does not line up well with native speaker fluency ratings. Therefore, either words per minute or syllables per minute (or second) are probably the most useful measures when working with non-native speakers. It is, however, important not to confuse this with syllables per second since syllable counts will always be higher than word counts. Incidentally, Tauroza and Allison (1990) did not find statistically significant differences when calculating rate by syllables per minute as opposed to words per minute. The calculation is fairly straightforward—simply count up all of the words or syllables uttered and divide by the number of seconds or minutes it took. When using a diagnostic passage, count the words or syllables in advance and use it with multiple clients to save time, but when using syllables, make sure to monitor for words such as *interested* that can be pronounced with a different number of syllables depending on dialect or idiolect.

## Pausing and Mean Length of Run (MLR)

One of the reasons that syllables or words per minute seems more valuable than articulatory rate is that much of what has a negative impact on our clients' naturalness and intelligibility relates to the length and frequency of pauses. Tromfimovich and Baker (2006) showed that both the frequency and duration of pauses were highly correlated with accentedness ratings, thus clinicians are well advised to monitor pauses, especially if they are lengthy, frequent, or at atypical boundaries (Kang, 2010). Mean length of run (MLR) is a way to measure the number of syllables produced in connected speech by determining the mean number of syllables between pauses. Grosjean and Deschamps (1975) found that native speakers averaged an MLR in spontaneous speech ranging from 7.42 to 14.85 depending on the type of task they were engaged in. In Hincks' study mentioned above, Swedish speakers produced MLRs that were 24% shorter when speaking English (L2) as opposed to their L1.

## Average Rate of Speech

Determining the average rate of speech for native speakers is challenging as there are a number of factors that determine rate, including dialect, idiolect, gender, age, and reading vs. speaking, among other variables, and there is contradictory data regarding all of them. For example, Butcher (1981) found an average of 6.13 syllables per second for reading while for spontaneous speech (either in reminiscing or retelling a story) it was 5.26, but Hewlett and Rendall (1998) found that conversation was faster than reading. Sandra Goetz (2013) states that researchers agree on an average rate of speech between

**Table 5–1.** Speech Rates

| Slow | Average | Fast |
|---|---|---|
| 90 words per minute | 180 words per minute | 240 words per minute |
| 2.0 syllables per second | 4.0 syllables per second | 5.3 syllables per second |

120 and 260 words per minute, but there is still quite a bit of variation reported in the literature. For example, Shipley and McCaffey's book *Assessment in Speech-Language Pathology* (2016) cites studies with reading and spontaneous speech ranges from 114 to 410 words per minute. It is easy to understand the large variance given the number of factors that can affect rate. Pimsleur, Hancock, and Furey (1977) reported an average rate of 177 words per minute for American radio announcers, and they discussed research showing that speakers average about 310 words per minute when asked to speak at their fastest possible intelligible rate. On a side note, Guiness World Records (Fastest recital of Hamlet's soliloquy) reports that Sean Shannon recited Hamlet's soliloquy in the "nunnery scene" at 655 words per minute!

Amee Shah, in her Comprehensive Assessment of Accentedness and Intelligibility (Shah, 2007) uses the following numbers to rate speakers: slow ± 180 syllables per minute, average = 180 to 260 syllables per minute, fast ± 260 syllables per minute, while Richard Cauldwell reports a set of ranges (shown in Table 5–1) in his book *Phonology for Listening* (2014).

The numbers in Table 5–1 are based on ranges, so average would be somewhere between the 120 to 220 range. SLPs should consider factors such as context, pragmatics, style, among countless others, to determine what is appropriate at any given point in treatment. While average speech rates provide some useful benchmarks for working with clients on their rate, the ultimate goal is to achieve clear and natural speech. Clinicians should be monitoring rate as much as possible, especially if it appears to be affecting intelligibility or naturalness. If clients need direct training, they can begin by developing an awareness of how their rate compares to native speakers, and they should be coached in how to self-monitor.

# Intonation

## The Big Picture

The second topic that should be addressed up front with clients is intonation. Of all the suprasegmentals, this is perhaps the most important because it is intertwined with so many other aspects of speech, and it has such awesome communicative power. While even clients at the beginning stages of English acquisition can benefit significantly from intonation training, for the most advanced speakers it often represents the final frontier as they seek to make subtle gains in their communication skills. When I began teaching TESOL pronunciation courses, I reserved this topic for the end because I realized how challenging it can be for non-natives, but over time I shifted it further toward the beginning because I saw that by addressing it early, it can be included as a part of all subsequent practice.

SLPs tend to favor the term *prosody* to *intonation*. There are two major ways to define intonation. A broad definition is essentially synonymous with suprasegmentals and includes rate, phrasing, and focus, while a narrow definition relates more specifically to the relevant pitch patterns at discourse level, and that is the definition used in this chapter. Whenever I ask a client to define intonation, they almost always take out their hand and wave it rhythmically while providing a definition. Intonation represents the music of speech, and clients have an intuitive sense of pitch changes and melody. If clients are unsure about intonation, I ask them to imagine listening to a conversation through a wall and how they would get a feel of the interaction that is occurring even if they cannot make out the individual sounds. You can also model a sentence with a great deal of pitch movement and then hum it to isolate the melody. While most clients have a general understanding of what intonation entails, they typically lack an understanding of how important a role it plays in communication. Because it is so abstract and variable, clients tend to take it for granted; they usually see the value in practicing a phoneme they are not producing accurately much more quickly than they appreciate work on their pitch patterns. Discussing intonation and providing clients with some background of its importance is a worthwhile investment. With some clients, half of the battle is convincing them of the need to change the pitch patterns of their speech.

As an illustration of the power of intonation, I ask clients to imagine their name being said by a parent, spouse, or child and to think of the different ways the segments of their name could be produced in a way that would make the meaning absolutely clear. Clients easily recognize that their loved ones can communicate thoughts such as affection, admiration, pride, or disappointment simply by varying their intonation. While the true communicative range of intonation is infinite, it can be helpful to focus on three major functions: grammar, meaning, and emotion. As an illustration, I often take a sentence such as "it's a beautiful day," and after saying it in a neutral manner, produce it as a question, then in a sarcastic way, and finally with a great deal of emotion. Clients can review the three versions and realize that we can use intonation to make a question, to change the meaning (in this case changing the meaning from "beautiful" to "terrible" through a sarcastic tone and body language), and finally we can emphasize our feelings by using pitch patterns to emote. I often share my experiences from graduate school working with clients who have aphasia following a left-hemispheric stroke. Two of the clients I worked with could only produce one or two different nonsense words, but they both had remarkably well-preserved intonation. When our right and left hemispheres are working together, language is shaped by both what we say and how we say it, and it is important for clients to understand the importance of both aspects.

Before working directly with intonation, there are several key concepts to consider, the first of which is understanding theories of intonation. Many efforts have been made to create something like an IPA system to categorize and explain intonation. There are two main schools of thought, with one focusing on tones and the other on contours, and there are a host of ideas about how to map out the music of speech. Anyone who delves into the literature regarding prosody is bound to be overwhelmed by the complexity of these competing viewpoints. There is probably no other discipline related to second language phonology where the gap between research and practice is so wide. While many researchers surely feel that practitioners do not provide an accurate theoretical framework to their clients, clinicians are justified in wondering whether these descriptive systems provide any benefit to clients seeking to become better communicators in a new language. Research in this area is evolving and at times contradictory, so systems that become ingrained in pronunciation materials often turn out to be of limited value for applied phonetics. For example, a system of three or four levels for English pitch first postulated in the 1940s is often used in the world of accent modification, but Dickerson (1989) has shown that native speakers pay more attention to whether something is stressed, as opposed to how much. Judy Gilbert, writing in *Pronunciation Myths* (Grant, 2014),  makes a good case for abandoning these types of descriptive systems as illustrated by the following anecdote: "in 1978, I complained to the professor of my Acoustic Phonetics course, John Ohala, that I was baffled by the four pitch-level system of intonation analysis. 'Why bother?' he said, casually, 'No one's paid any attention to Trager-Smith for twenty years.' This little exchange demonstrated the difference between his world of advanced research and my own world as an English as a second language (ESL) teacher. It was clear that in *my* world, at *that* time, people did indeed pay attention to Trager-Smith; the analysis system was simply accepted as factual. My objection was a practical one: If I couldn't understand it, how could I teach it? Professor Ohala's remark, however, suggested a second objection to the approach: perhaps the analysis itself was unsound." Clinicians should use their judgment to determine whether any type of visual framework will help clients achieve more natural intonation, but a good case can be made for focusing on very basic descriptions and providing good modeling. While the range of intonation can be daunting, clinicians should feel confident that they can rely on their own sense of what is natural when shaping clients' speech.

A second important aspect related to research is that we need to be careful about making conclusive statements about connections between any intonation patterns and communicative functions. Clients should be trained to develop an ear for intonation and to become adept at analyzing and imitating it, but they need to know that there are virtually no absolutes when it comes to these suprasegmentals. For example, clinicians might be tempted to tell clients that they need to use rising pitch whenever they make "wh" questions, but the results of corpus linguistics research analyzing the percent of "wh" questions which are rising has ranged from about 50 to 90%, not the expected 100% (Hedberg, Sosa, & Görgülü, 2014). Intonation is incredibly complex, and the truth is that there is no absolute relationship between any pitch pattern and a particular grammatical, semantic, or paralinguistic element of communication. This is why intonation can be so challenging for clinicians and clients, but by understanding this, we can work on developing practical and realistic goals for developing awareness. Intonation is simply too powerful to be put in a box, but once clients learn to appreciate its beauty, they can gain confidence in using it to their advantage.

A third element that is essential to discuss with clients is the possible interference of their L1 intonation patterns (and communication styles) in their ability to convey messages in English. The pitch patterns of a language vary by dialect, age, gender, and many other factors, and they are in constant flux. Because of this, it is no surprise that the intonation patterns of two languages are usually very different. These patterns are so ingrained that clients are often unaware of when they are using intonation that sounds different from the patterns used by native speakers of English. As an example, we can consider a speaker of Japanese making a statement such as "I just won the lottery." Because there is less pitch movement in Japanese, an English speaker might be taken aback by the lack of excitement and might even expect that there was some kind of problem instead of a fortunate event. A speaker of Italian, on the other hand, might make a simple statement such as "I'm going to the store," but because the pitch patterns in that language are relatively dynamic compared to English, it might sound overly excited. Clients need to know that these cultural patterns in the way they speak may interfere with the message they are trying to convey. Discussing intonation presents a good opportunity to highlight some of the nonlinguistic factors that play a role in communication. Accent training should involve not just what comes out of clients' mouths, but also their facial expressions and gestures. These factors should always form a crucial part of any work on intonation since they often go hand in hand with prosody to shape meaning.

The goal of intonation training should therefore focus on developing awareness. It is true that non-native speakers who have spent longer amounts of time in an English-speaking environment will slowly absorb the intonation patterns around them, but accent modification is an effective way of speeding this process up considerably. When we work on segmentals, we can focus on a clearly defined target and practice producing the same consonant or vowel until it is accurate, but intonation is much more abstract. While we will not be able to give clients a precise blueprint concerning the pitch patterns of English, there are several ways to raise consciousness. Perhaps one of the most useful means of fostering change is to try to encapsulate the biggest global difference between the client's intonation and that of English and draw their attention to it. For example, if a client's speech sounds monotonous, they can concentrate on producing wider pitch variations. Often, these overarching targets help clients home in on the most salient differences. They should also spend some time reviewing particular patterns to build awareness. It is essential to point out that these are not set in stone; native speakers play with intonation constantly, and they are incredibly imaginative with it. It would be a disservice to imply that there is one way to produce the pitch pattern for any message, grammatical structure, or emotion in English, but by highlighting some typical patterns, we can raise consciousness.

## Typical Intonation Patterns

Since the true range of intonation is essentially limitless, it may help to provide clients with some scaffolding in the form of typical intonation patterns. Some of the more easily defined samples, as outlined below, can help them develop some awareness. It is always worth reminding clients about the range of variability and creativity involved in discourse.

### End of a Statement

In most statements, English speakers reduce pitch at the very end to let the listener know that they are finished with the statement. They also tend to put some stress on the last content word of the last phrase before they come down, but we will look at that in some more detail later. When most speakers say a sentence such as "I just got a new job," the word *job* will jump out because its pitch will come out relatively high and then drop. If non-natives do not use this type of pattern, they may sound unnatural because listeners will wait for them to finish their thought. It may help build awareness by demonstrating that some speakers of American English (usually young women) use a high rising terminal pitch pattern, but this is often mildly stigmatized. The clinician can train the expected pattern by providing models of both types and having the client decide whether it marks a completed sentence or not as illustrated in the sample exercise below.

Listen to the following sentences and decide if they are finished or not:

1. I've been doing some yoga
2. She went to the police department and filed a report
3. We are expecting them to bring chips, and salsa
4. They didn't want to go downtown for the concert
5. Let's go to Frank's house, and then to the restaurant

### Question Intonation

In theory, when we use "wh" questions, we tend to go down in pitch, and when we ask yes/no questions, we tend to go up. Although this is often presented as obligatory, these are just tendencies, so you will find many cases where this is not true. The key for clients is to develop familiarity with this pattern, and then monitor for natural variations. Remember that in English we can make yes/no questions by changing word order, or by changing intonation, while in many languages, intonation is the only possible way to make a question. In English, creating a question by changing intonation is actually very common, and is the first kind of question marker that children learn. Intonation can also express disbelief or surprise. Creating a distinction between question and surprise can be challenging for clients, and it is an excellent opportunity to teach your client to include facial expressions and more subtle differences in timing and phrasing. Table 5–2 illustrates an activity that can be used to target statement, question, and doubt intonation patterns.

**Table 5–2.** Statements, Questions, and Doubts

Read each phrase as a statement, question, or statement of disbelief. Your partner will then identify which intonation you used.

| Sentence | Statement↘ | Question↗ | Doubt↗ |
|---|---|---|---|
| 1. He lives in India | | | |
| 2. You haven't done it yet | | | |
| 3. It costs $99 | | | |
| 4. It looks like it will rain | | | |
| 5. Things are getting better | | | |
| 6. We shouldn't do that again | | | |
| 7. We have the same last name | | | |
| 8. They're going to have to do it over | | | |
| 9. He won't be able to finish on time | | | |
| 10. He doesn't know how to drive | | | |

## List Intonation

In much the same way as we conclude a neutral statement, we tell listeners that we are finished with a list by coming down sharply on the last item. We rise on all of the items preceding the final one.

I'll bring pizza, beer, donuts, wine, and pretzels.

You can often tell which one is the last item if it is the only one preceded by *and*, but this won't always work, so intonation is the best clue. The following is a sample exercise. Come down on the last item in each list:

1. She bought lettuce, and tomatoes, and pickles.
2. To make tacos you need meat, cheese, tomatoes, shells.
3. I've been to Korea, Thailand, and Japan.
4. They'll need money, food, clothing.
5. He can speak Norwegian, Danish, Swedish, and German.

## Choice Questions

If we take a sentence such as, "Would you like beer or wine?" we can actually produce it in several distinct ways to indicate different types of questions. If we go up on *beer* and then

**Table 5–3.** Yes/No and Choice Questions

| Sentence | Choice ↗↘ | Yes/No ↗ |
|---|---|---|
| 1. Are you coming Friday or Saturday? | | |
| 2. Can you meet us at 8 or 9? | | |
| 3. Would you like beer or wine? | | |
| 4. Are you going to Spain or Portugal? | | |
| 5. Did you live in Australia or New Zealand? | | |
| 6. Do you like classical music or ballet? | | |
| 7. Does your last name begin with a *v* or a *w*? | | |
| 8. Can he drive a car or a motorcycle? | | |
| 9. Does it usually rain in April or May? | | |
| 10. Was he driving 60 or 70 miles per hour? | | |

come down on *wine*, it is a choice question, and the listener answers either "beer" or "win*e*." Going up after the last item makes it a yes/no question and the listener isn't deciding between two offerings. In this case, the answer might be a simple "yes" or "no." Finally, if you don't come down at all, your intonation will signal that it is an unfinished list, implying that there are even more options available. Table 5–3 is an example of an activity that can be used to target the production and perception of these two intonation patterns.

## Tag Questions

We often use tag questions (i.e., didn't you? wasn't it?) after a statement. There are two basic patterns. With the example sentence, "You've done this before, haven't you?" if we go up in pitch at the end, we are asking a real question, or we are unsure about the statement, and we often expect an answer. If we step down in pitch at the end, then we are just confirming the statement. It is not a real question, and we do not expect an answer. This is really just a way to involve the listener in the conversation. Generally, this type of intonation pattern is more common, but it is also difficult for many non-native speakers, especially those who speak Romance languages, and they frequently need more work on the confirmation pattern than on any other intonation pattern. An example of an activity that can be used to help clients identify and produce both types of intonations is outlined in Table 5–4.

## Emphasis

In theory we can put stress on any word in a sentence, and there are many reasons to shift stress depending on context. Here are a few examples:

**Table 5–4.** Tag Questions

| Sentence | Confirmation ↘ | Real Question ↗ |
|---|---|---|
| 1. Your name's George, isn't it? | | |
| 2. It's going to rain tomorrow, isn't it? | | |
| 3. You wanted to go, didn't you? | | |
| 4. We should offer to help, shouldn't we? | | |
| 5. He didn't do it, did he? | | |
| 6. She's never done it before, has she? | | |
| 7. We're late, aren't we? | | |
| 8. Berlin is the capital of Germany, isn't it? | | |
| 9. There's enough room, isn't there? | | |
| 10. It's over, isn't it? | | |

To answer a question: Who went to the store? **I** went to the store.

To correct information: A: She got married in 1998. B: No, it was 199**7**.

To agree with someone: A: He plays guitar really well. B: He **does** play guitar well!

Stress will be covered in detail in a later section on prosody, but clients should be made aware of it at an early stage in training since they are likely to produce sentences that may be possible in certain, but not all contexts.

### *Question Word Intonation*

Look at the following dialogs:

> A: He lives in Spain.
> B: Where?
> A: Spain

> A: He lives in Spain.
> B: Where?
> A: Madrid

Although they look the same on the page, the answers tell you that they use different intonation. Rising intonation means "Where did you say he lives,?" ("I didn't hear you," or "I can't believe it") and falling intonation means "Where in Spain does he live?"

### Rhetorical Questions

When we ask questions we already know the answer to, we use another intonation pattern, which is often used as a technique during presentations.

Example: And how long have we been providing specialized delivery services to businesses throughout the country? We've been on the job for over 30 years.

### Parentheticals

We use a special pattern when we are adding extra information in the middle of a sentence. We often call these parentheticals because the sentence will still make sense if you take out the added information.

Example: My father, who just retired last year, loves to play golf whenever he can.

Note that *My father loves to play golf whenever he can* is also a complete sentence.

## Activities to Develop Intonation Awareness

It is recommended that the conversation about intonation begin early because these patterns will be such an important part of all further accent work; any investment up front is bound to pay off later. Essentially, clients practice intonation every time they speak during a session, so there are always opportunities to spot-check any patterns that do not sound natural or that convey the wrong message. It is also useful to work directly on intonation at times, and the possibilities for creative activities are limitless.

Clients can practice producing vowels in isolation when provided prompts, focusing on varying their intonation to provide a natural response. This type of activity is very effective at showing the power of intonation when no real words are being spoken.

Example: Respond to each statement with the word *oh* /oʊ/:

1. I guess I'm going to need to borrow some money from you.
2. He lost the race by half a second!
3. She says she's much better at that than you are.
4. So they decided to cancel the wedding.

Appendix 5–2 provides more samples of this type of activity to use with clients. A similar activity uses words or phrases with some guidance about the context or speaker's intent. For example:

Say the sentence "It was OK," in the following ways:

1. about something that was surprisingly good,
2. about something that was average,

3. about something that is no longer OK, and

4. with disbelief.

These activities are excellent ways to highlight the fact that certain words are extremely intonation dependent. The meaning of *OK* can range (at a minimum) from *not very good* to *great*, depending on how it is said. Appendix 5–3 provides more sample prompts.

Appendix 5–4 is a variation on this activity. The client is given a list of adjectives such as *bored, excited, sad,* and *surprised* and some sentences such as "It's time to go." The client then produces the sentence with one of the emotions indicated and the clinician guesses the intended adjective. Since the client does not state in advance which adjective was chosen, the clinician can more objectively evaluate the client's ability to convey the emotion.

A clever idea that first appeared in an article by Allen (1971) is the use of single word dialogs. Although this activity works best with two clients, it is also possible for the clinician to play one role and assign the client the other. The dialogs consist of single words, but they only make sense if appropriate intonation patterns are used. An example might look like this:

Leftovers

A: Dinner

B: Ready

A: What

B: Leftovers

A: Leftovers

B: Leftovers

A: Again

B: Again

A: OK

B: Good

Appendix 5–5 contains several more examples. Short dialogs of any kind are also highly effective, and one interesting way to approach these with the client is to develop two different ways to say the same dialog. In the following dialog, taken from Appendix 5–6, there might be one version where *funny* means *humorous,* and then another version in which it means *odd.*

A. Your friend Don is really funny.

B. What do you mean?

A. I think you know what I mean. How long have you known him?

B. Just a couple of years.

Clinicians can train clients in shadowing techniques during which they listen to samples of native speech and then repeat what is said just a split second afterwards.

They can have a script of the text, but instead of reading along at exactly the same time, there is a slight delay to allow the client to mimic the speaker's intonation pattern. This technique is popular in Japan, especially to train simultaneous interpreters, and it has shown some signs of promise (Foote & McDonough, 2017), although it presents challenges because of the cognitive demands it places on learners. A similar technique that is probably more suited for accent modification conducted by SLPs is called *mirroring* (Meyers, 2013, 2014). In this case, clients choose a 1 to 2-minute English video sample featuring a proficient speaker of their L1 who can serve as a good pronunciation model for them. The clinician should vet the sample and discuss the client's reason for choosing it. Both client and clinician should analyze the suprasegmental features and body language of the speaker for awareness building, and then the client practices and prepares a video imitating the speaker as closely as possible. After some feedback and discussion, the client practices some more and rerecords the video. Role plays are very effective for working on intonation as well, and Appendix 5–7 offers samples of two- and three-person role plays for use in pairs and groups. Real differences in intonation patterns often emerge during this type of activity. Role plays are also sometimes helpful in working with clients who are hesitant to use more dynamic patterns in their speech, because the roles can encourage clients to adopt a character. There is really no limit to the types of activities that can help clients produce more natural sounding prosody, and clients and clinicians can explore ideas that are both productive and fun.

# References

Allen, V. F. (1971). Teaching intonation: From theory to practice. *TESOL Quarterly, 5*(1), 73–81.

Anderson-Hsieh, J., & Venkatagiri, H. (1994). Syllable duration and pausing in the speech of intermediate and high proficiency Chinese ESL speakers. *TESOL Quarterly, 28*, 807–812.

Butcher, A. (1981). *Aspects of the speech pause: Phonetic correlates and communicative functions*. Kiel, West Germany: Institut für Phonetik der Universität.

Cauldwell, R. (2007). Defining fluency for air traffic control. *Speak Out. 37*, 10–16.

Cauldwell, R. (2014). *Phonology for listening: Teaching the stream of speech*. Speech in Action, Birmingham, UK.

Derwing, T. M., Rossiter, M. J., Munro, M. J., & Thomson, R. I. (2004). Second language fluency: Judgments on different tasks. *Language Learning, 54*(4), 655–679.

Dickerson, W. B. (1989). *Stress in the speech stream: The rhythm of spoken English*. Urbana, IL: University of Illinois Press.

Fastest recital of Hamlet's soliloquy. Retrieved from: http://www.guinnessworldrecords.com /world-records/67539-fastest-recital-of-hamlets -soliloquy

Foote, J., & Mcdonough, K. (2017). Using shadowing with mobile technology to improve L2 pronunciation. *Journal of Second Language Pronunciation. 3*, 34–56.

Fries, C. (1943). *Intensive course in English for Latin-American students*. (Vols. 1–4). Ann Arbor: The University of Michigan Press.

Goetz, S. (2013). *Fluency in native and nonnative English speech*. Amsterdam, The Netherlands: Benjamins.

Grant, L. J. (2014). *Pronunciation myths: Applying second language research to classroom teaching*. Ann Arbor, MI: University of Michigan Press.

Grosjean, F., & Deschamps, A. (1975). Analyse contrastive des variables temporelles de l'anglais et du français: Vitesse de parole et variables composantes, phénomènes d'hésitation. *Phonetica, 31*, 144–184

Hedberg, N., Sosa, J., & Görgülü, E. (2014). The meaning of intonation in yes-no questions in American English: A corpus study. *Corpus Linguistics and Linguistic Theory, 13*(2), 321–368.

Hewlett, N., & Rendall, M. (1998). Rural versus urban accent as an influence on the rate of speech. *Journal of the International Phonetic Association. 28*, 63–71.

Hincks, R., (2010) Speaking rate and information content in English lingua franca oral presentations. *English for Specific Purposes, 29*(1), 4–18.

Jacewicz, E., Fox, R. A., O'Neill, C., & Salmons, J. (2009). Articulation rate across dialect, age, and gender. *Language Variation and Change, 21*(2), 233–256.

Kang, O. (2010). Suprasegmental features that contribute most to listeners' judgments of L2 comprehensibility and accent. *System, 38*, 301–315.

Meyers, C. (2013). Mirroring project update: Intelligible accented speakers as pronunciation models. *TESOL Video News*. Retrieved from http://newsmanager.commpartners.com/te solvdmis/issues/2013-07-27/6.html

Meyers, C. (2014). Intelligible accented speakers as pronunciation models. In J. Levis & S. Mc-Crocklin (Eds.). *Proceedings of the 5th annual conference of pronunciation in second language learning and teaching (PSLLT;* pp. 172–76). Ames, IA: Iowa State University.

Munro, M. J., & Derwing, T. M. (1998). The effects of speaking rate on listener evaluations of native and foreign-accented speech. *Language Learning, 48*, 159–182.

Pimsleur, P., Hancock, C., & Furey, P. (1977). Speech rate and listening comprehension. In M. K. Burt, H. C. Dulay, & M. Finocchiaro (Eds.), *Viewpoints on English as a second language* (pp. 27–34). New York: Regents.

Polyanskaya, L., Ordin, M., & Busa, M. G. (2017). Relative salience of speech rhythm and speech rate on perceived foreign accent in a second language. *Language and Speech 60*(3), 333–355.

Shah, A. P. (2007). *Comprehensive Assessment of Accentedness and Intelligibility (CAAI)* [Assessment instrument]. Cleveland, OH: EBAM Institute.

Shipley, K. G., & MacAfee, J. G. (2016). *Assessment in speech-language pathology: A resource manual.* Boston, MA, USA: Cengage Learning.

Tauroza, S., & Allison, D. (1990). Speech rates in British English, *Applied Linguistics, 11*, 90–105.

Trofimovich, P., & Baker, W. (2006). Learning second-language suprasegmentals: Effect of L2 experience on prosody and fluency characteristics of L2 speech. *Studies in Second Language Acquisition, 28*, 1–30

# 5–1

# Sample Worksheet: Sounds and Patterns

**Sounds** are like the bricks, and **patterns** are like the architecture of language.
A. Read the descriptions of some pronunciation problems. Are they problems at the sound or pattern level?

1. Kash has problems making the /w/ and it often sounds like /v/. When he says "why" it sounds like "vie."

2. Tan says the /s/ and /d/ sounds at the beginning of a word, but she often leaves them off at the end of a word, so *dialed* sounds like *dial*.

3. Rajiv sometimes forgets where to put the stress in a word.

4. Toshi has real problems hearing the difference between /r/ and /l/. The words *right* and *light* sound the same to him.

5. Chen does not connect words when he speaks, so many Americans tell him that his speech sounds choppy.

6. Many people tell Abdul that they can't understand him because he speaks too quickly.

7. Nicole has problems with her vowels, so *buddy* and *body* sound the same.

8. Yvonne usually says /z/ in words that begin with *th* /ð/. She says, "I went to ze store."

9. When In-Sook uses question tags like "It's a nice day, isn't it?" many Americans aren't sure if she's asking a question or making a statement.

10. Fernando can't make the /z/, so "zoo" sounds like "Sue."

# 5-2

# Intonation and Vowels Worksheet

Use appropriate intonation for each vowel sound in response to the sentences you hear:

1. *ah* /ɑ/
   a. Look at the new puppy I just bought!
   b. So after all that work preparing for the interview, I didn't get the job.
   c. See? You just have to punch in this code, and it works great.
   d. We had to watch a dissection in class today.

2. *ooh* /u/
   a. Did you see what just happened to that guy?
   b. And when I walked in, they were kissing!
   c. Didn't you remember that we have a meeting with the boss right now?
   d. Would you like some fresh-baked pie?

3. *oh* /oʊ/
   a. I guess I'm going to need to borrow some money from you.
   b. He lost the race by half a second!
   c. She says she's much better at that than you are.
   d. So they decided to cancel the wedding.

4. *uh* /ʌ/
   a. Isn't that my seat?
   b. Why did you come home so late last night?
   c. Didn't you have something to tell me?
   d. I think I should probably handle this.

# 5-3

# Intonation Practice Worksheet

Read each word or phrase in bold the way you might say it in situations a-d:

1. **"Hello"**
   a. to a friend you see every day
   b. to a friend you haven't seen for 3 years
   c. to a 6-month old baby
   d. to someone you caught doing something bad

2. **"How are you doing?"**
   a. to someone you haven't seen for 20 years
   b. to someone who has recently lost a member of the family
   c. after someone asked you how you were doing
   d. to a neighbor that you don't like.

3. **"I never go to bars."**
   a. by a person that totally disapproves of drinking alcohol
   b. said sarcastically by someone who always goes to bars
   c. said before: ". . . but I really like going out to dance."
   d. said before: ". . . but my friends do."

4. **"You're a terrific tennis player."**
   a. neutral
   b. said with disbelief
   c. sarcastic, after your tennis partner missed a shot
   d. said before "but a terrible golfer."

5. **"What are you doing?"**
   a. neutral
   b. disapproving (as if to say, "You shouldn't be doing that.")
   c. repeat what you said, as if you didn't hear the answer—
   d. challenging, (as if to say, "I'm not going to answer your question until you answer mine!")

6. **"You put that down."**
   a. to a misbehaving child
   b. after someone mistakenly put something up
   c. questioningly, after someone told you what they wrote on a test
   d. disbelievingly, as if you can't believe your friend put that down

7. **"It was OK"**
   a. about something that was surprisingly good
   b. about something that was average
   c. about something that is no longer OK
   d. said with disbelief

# 5–4

# An Intonation Game

neutral          bored                 angry          sad
sarcastic        disapproving          doubtful       happy

Pick a sentence below and read it using intonation suggesting one of the adjectives above:

1. He's never done that before.
2. She did it very fast.
3. He loves her.
4. They live in that old house.
5. It's time to go.
6. We hate that.
7. He has no friends.
8. I missed it.

# 5-5

# Intonation Conversations Worksheet

1. **Leftovers**

   A: Dinner

   B: Ready

   A: What

   B: Leftovers

   A: Leftovers

   B: Leftovers

   A: Again

   B: Again

   A: OK

   B: Good

2. **On the Train**

   A: Tickets

   B: Pardon

   A: Tickets

   B: Tickets

   A: Now

   B: OK

   A: Well

   B: Wait

   A: Hurry

B: Here

A: Thanks

3. **The Escape**

A: When

B: Tomorrow

A: Tomorrow

B: Right

A: What time

B: What time

A: Right

B: Eleven

A: Chances

B: Good

A: Dangerous

B: Maybe

A: Tomorrow

B: Tomorrow

# 5-6

# Short Dialogs Worksheet

Practice saying each dialog with two different intonations:

1. **A.** The homework assignment is due tomorrow.

   **B.** Now you tell me.

   **A.** Well, have you done it yet?

   **B.** I'm working on it.

2. **A.** Where were you?

   **B.** Out with some friends.

   **A.** And you probably didn't have time to call me.

   **B.** Yeah. I guess not.

3. **A.** I really need your help with this.

   **B.** Well, I'm actually kind of busy.

   **A.** Are you sure you can't spare just a minute or two?

   **B.** Okay.

4. **A.** Can you please step inside?

   **B.** Did you need to see me about something?

   **A.** I sure did. Have a seat.

   **B.** It sounds important.

   **A.** Well, have a look at this.

   **B.** Oh. I see.

5. **A.** I've got something to tell you.

   **B.** Okay. I'm all ears.

   **A.** Well, I've been meaning to tell you for quite a while.

   **B.** Well, you might as well get it off your chest.

6.  **A.** Your friend Don is really funny.

    **B.** What do you mean?

    **A.** I think you know what I mean. How long have you known him?

    **B.** Just a couple of years.

7.  **A.** How's that new restaurant?

    **B.** Okay.

    **A.** Because I was thinking of trying it out.

    **B.** You were?

8.  **A.** Time to go.

    **B.** Coming.

    **A.** Did you hear me?

    **B.** I said I was coming.

# 5-7

# Intonation Role Plays

**Congratulations!** (2-person role play)

*(Two people are sitting in in a bar.)*

A: Hey! Over here!

B: (Comes over) Hey! Long time no see! What have you been up to lately?

A: Not much, that's for sure. And you?

B: Well, I guess I do have some pretty big news.

A: Come on, the suspense is killing me.

B: No, really. What have you been doing these past few weeks? The last time I saw you, you were going to look for a new job.

A: Well, I didn't have to. I was offered a new position in the accounting department.

B: A step up in the big business world!

A: I wouldn't exaggerate, but I'm pleased.

B: I hear you. That's great! I hope the money's better!

A: I can't complain. Now, enough about me. I'm dying to hear your news.

B: Well . . . I'm getting married!

A: NO! You said you'd never get married. I can't believe it.

B: Well that was then and this is now. You've got to meet my fiancé.

A: So come on. This is all news to me. I didn't even know you were dating.

B: We weren't. We've just been dating for two weeks now.

A: . . . and you're getting married?!

B: I know, I know. I can't help it. I'm just completely head over heels in love.

A: Well, congratulations! That is fantastic! This calls for a toast!

B: Thanks! I'm glad to hear you feel that way. I thought you might think I was crazy.

A: You? Crazy? Nah!

B: Bartender! I think my friend here is ready to buy me a drink.

**Waiting** (3-person role play)

*(Husband and wife are waiting at Joe's Bar and Grill; later, server enters.)*

Husband: We've been waiting for more than 30 minutes!

Wife: Terry, are you sure you read the directions correctly?

Husband: Do you think I made a mistake?! I'm sure he said Joe's Bar and Grill.

Wife: I wish you'd brought the directions with you.

Husband: It's no use worrying about that now. Anyway, let's concentrate on what we'll be doing this time tomorrow? I'm so excited about getting away from it all.

Wife: So am I. Just think, this time tomorrow we'll be lying on the beach soaking up the sun, and then you'll buy me lunch at the most expensive restaurant in town.

Husband: Whatever . . . (pause). Anyway, I wish he'd get here. And speaking of food, I'm getting hungry!

Wife: Why don't you ask our server for help?

Husband: OK. (*goes up to the server*) Excuse me, we've been waiting for over a half an hour for a friend. Have you seen anyone looking for somebody?

Server: Look, I'm a little busy. Did you want to order another round of drinks or not?

Husband: Thanks for the great service. I just don't understand. Our friend Alex is never late.

Server: Well, maybe he's at Joe's Bar.

Husband: It's a *she* actually. And did you say Joe's *Bar*? I thought this *was* Joe's Bar.

Server: This is Joe's Bar and *Grill*. She's probably at Joe's *Bar*. That's downtown.

Husband: Do you think you could call over there and see if she's there?

Server: No problem. Maybe I can just take an hour off work to drive over and look for her.

Husband: And maybe we'll forget about leaving you a tip.

Server: All right already! I get your point. I'll call. (*telephoning*) Yes, this is Joe's Bar and Grill. Is there an Alex waiting there? A woman named Alex I should say . . . (*he waits for the other person to ask for Alex*) Yes, great. Thanks. Goodbye.

Husband: She's there, isn't she?

Server: Yes, she's there and she's been waiting for half an hour.

Husband: Oh, no! She is at Joe's Bar! Is there a taxi nearby?

Server: How am I supposed to know? Why don't you try looking outside, Einstein!

Husband: Let's go! The service here is simply wonderful.

Wife: And your ability to follow directions is even more wonderful.

Server: Wow, what a lovely couple!

# 6

# Consonants

## Working with Consonants

### Familiar Ground

Therapy aimed at improving the accuracy of consonants lies at the very heart of speech-language pathology and goes back to the beginnings of our profession. This is generally the aspect of accent modification that comes the easiest to clinicians entering the field, and if anything, the danger is that clinicians may focus on consonants at the expense of work on the vowels or suprasegmentals, which often have greater impact on intelligibility and naturalness. Most SLPs have a good grounding in the classification of consonants and how to elicit them. This chapter provides a brief overview of the consonants of English, but it is intended to supplement, rather than replace, a good phonetics textbook or articulation drill manual. The goal is to review the aspects of consonants that are most important for working with non-native speakers, and to provide some practical tips on how to get results with clients. It can be useful to give clients a cursory review of all of the consonants as a means of demystifying our sound system, but clients typically present with several especially problematic phonemes that can be shaped through training.

### Classification of Consonants

Consonants are defined as speech sounds produced with relatively restricted airflow. Although most clients can identify whether a sound is a consonant or vowel easily, depending on their language and country of origin, they may have difficulty providing more detail about the articulatory mechanics involved in producing them. Place, manner, and voicing serve as the major distinguishing features of consonants and will most likely be the most helpful way of explaining their production to clients. Table 6–1 is adapted from the IPA chart (International Phonetic Association, 2014) and should provide enough

**Table 6–1.** Classification of English Consonants

| | Bilabial (made with lips) | Labio-dental (lips and teeth) | Dental (teeth) | Alveolar (gum ridge) | Post-alveolar (behind gum ridge) | Palatal (roof of mouth) | Velar (soft palate) | Glottal (vocal cords) |
|---|---|---|---|---|---|---|---|---|
| stop | p b | | | t d | | | k g | |
| affricate | | | | | tʃ dʒ | | | |
| nasal | m | | | n | | | ŋ | |
| fricative | | f v | θ ð | s z | ʃ ʒ | | | h |
| approximant | w | | | ɹ | | j | w | |
| lateral approximant | | | | l | | | | |

level of detail to outline the consonant inventory of English in a way that is meaningful for clients.

This type of chart helps clients visualize the sounds of English, but clinicians should provide clients with one that shows all of the phonemes of English with sample words. In terms of place, the English consonants are produced from the lips to the vocal folds, with the most common site being the alveolar ridge. The /w/ is listed under two columns on this chart to represent its two places of production; the IPA chart (International Phonetic Association, 2014) lists it in the Other Symbols section as a voiced labial-velar approximant. As a general rule, clinicians can focus on whatever information is most relevant to clients, so this sound can simply be called bilabial. The places of articulation are indicated by column and the manners of production are indicated by row. While the IPA chart does not feature a row for affricates, clinicians should add a row to include the two found in English. For consonants that have unvoiced and voiced versions, the voiceless phoneme occupies the first space in each box, and the voiced version follows to the right. This chart focuses on the consonant phonemes of English, and the allophones such as /ɾ,ʔ,ŋ̩/ will be addressed later. By focusing on the phonemes, the priority is on intelligibility, and when working with the allophones, the intent is to help the client sound more natural.

## Consonants of the World

As shown in Table 6–1, English has 24 consonant phonemes, which places it in the average range in a study of the consonant inventories of the world's languages by the World Atlas of Language Structures (Dryer & Haspelmath, 2013) in which the mean number of consonant phonemes was 22.7 and the median was 21. The consonant inventories of the

566 languages analyzed ranged from 6–122, and they were divided into the following categories: small (6–14), moderately small (15–18), average (19–25), moderately large (26–33), and large (34 or more consonants). Peter Ladefoged (2005) estimated the total number of consonants in the world to be 600. By comparing a chart from the Languages of the World website (Pereltsvaig), representing the most common consonants of the world, with the phonemic inventory of English, we can see that the following English consonants can be considered relatively rare: /θ,ð,z,ʒ,ɹ/. Note that while both /z/ and /ʒ/ are rare, their voiceless counterparts /s/ and /ʃ/, respectively, are relatively common, so it is likely that clients will produce those devoiced versions as substitutions. In the case of the /ɹ/, clients' languages often feature an /r/, which will easily be recognized by English speakers and will be a suitable substitute in terms of intelligibility. In contrast, the /θ,ð/ pair is a set of phonemes that does not have an analogous phoneme in most clients' languages. These sounds occur in just 7.3% of the languages in the World Atlas study (Dryer & Haspelmath, 2013), and in terms of the languages spoken by typical accent modification clients in the United States, they probably represent an even lower percentage, with Iberian Spanish and Greek being two languages featuring them that come to mind. Pereltsvaig's chart does not list affricates, so we can add the two in our language /ʧ, ʤ/ to the list, with /ʤ/ generally presenting more of a challenge for our clients.

## Client Awareness

### The Basics

In most cases, clinicians should provide clients with an overview of the consonants before targeting the phonemes which are giving them difficulty. Although clinicians can skip this stage and get right to work on articulation practice, a 5 to 10-minute overview of the consonants is likely to pay off by increasing overall awareness. A good place to start is an orientation of where the articulators are located, and a sagittal diagram can help the client visualize the anatomy involved. This is also a good opportunity to provide some training in the anatomical names that you will use during the sessions. Everyday language is preferable to technical jargon, and the Table 6–2 provides examples of some

**Table 6–2.** Terminology

| Technical Name | Client-Friendly Terminology |
|---|---|
| Alveolar ridge | Gum ridge |
| Palate | Roof of the mouth |
| Velum | Soft palate |
| Larynx | Voice box |
| Nasal cavity | Nose |

options for terminology, depending on the client's level of English and familiarity with linguistics.

After explaining the terminology, clinicians can verify clients' understanding using simple diagrams to elicit the names of the major articulators before embarking on a review of how the consonants are produced. Once clients can identify the major articulators, clinicians should point out some of the anatomical features they may be less familiar with, such as the alveolar ridge. Clinicians can also review the basic physiology of speech. Children learn their native phonologies implicitly, without direct instruction, so adults typically have limited understanding of how speech sounds are actually produced. While clients generally have good proprioception when it comes to their lips and jaw, for example, they usually have limited awareness of how their tongue articulates with the alveolar ridge, palate, and velum. In addition, depending on country of origin, clients may not understand phonation and its role in speech production. As an awareness building exercise, clinicians should walk clients through a series of consonants and elicit information about place, manner, or voicing. Clinicians can model selected sounds and have the client describe how to make them, or use a simple worksheet, such as that in Appendix 6–1, to provide more structure.

When providing an overview of the categorization of consonants, a suggested order would be place, manner, and then voicing. After clients have had some exposure to the place of articulation for several of the consonant phonemes (preferably basic ones, such as stops), they can review the manner for each. Clients should already be familiar with stop consonants, and their language will likely have some fricatives, but it may not have affricates, or if it does, they may be allophonic and not contrast with their homorganic fricatives. As a part of the overview, clinicians can highlight the difference between a stop such as /t/, a fricative such as /ʃ/, and an affricate such as /tʃ/. A good starting point is to make sure clients understand which of the three types of sounds can be produced continuously (/ʃ/) and which ones can only be repeated in rapid succession but not as a continuous sounds (/t, tʃ/). Clinicians can use their judgment as to the level of technical terminology they use, but a good rule of thumb is to use the minimal amount necessary to get results.

### Voicing

To illustrate voicing, clinicians can model the /s/ and /z/ fricatives and ask clients to explain what distinguishes them. Fricatives are always the best starting point to address voicing since they are continuous and the difference between voiced and voiceless fricatives is salient. If clients guess that there are changes taking place above the glottis, the clinician places a hand just above the larynx and alternates between the two sounds, explaining that no changes are taking place above the hand. With this scaffolding, clients can be guided to focus on the difference in phonation. Stops in English are distinguished by other factors such as aspiration and vowel lengthening, so clients should not attempt to determine whether they are voiced or not by sounding them out or saying English words. It is important to have clients feel their faces when they produce the voiced phonemes so they can sense the vibration at their vocal folds and in their entire vocal tract. Some clients will have a basic understanding of voicing and may even know which English consonants are voiced, but for those who do not encourage them to practice identifying the fricatives and to memorize the stops. Clients are often surprised to discover how important the voicing distinction is in several aspects of English pronunciation, such as vowel length and the assimilation of endings, so it is definitely a worthwhile investment for them to sort the consonants into these two categories quickly. Clinicians need to have an idea about the phonemic inventory of a client's language to determine whether voicing is likely to present problems. Spanish, for example, does not use voiced fricatives phonemically. Appendix 6–2 features minimal pairs to illustrate some differences in voicing.

### Nasals, Liquids, and Approximants

Nasals are relatively easy to demonstrate by asking clients to produce words that end in /m, n, ŋ/ and then hold the final sound. While holding the nasal, clinicians can instruct clients to pinch their noses to help them realize that the air is flowing through the nasal cavity. Generally, /m/ and /n/ will provide few challenges for clients, but there are some noticeable exceptions, such as the Sichuan dialect of Mandarin, where /n/ and /l/ are considered to be in free variation, and clients may alternate them. There may also be phonotactic constraints in some languages on /m,n/, especially in final position. In contrast, /ŋ/ tends to present more issues for clients and they will typically substitute an /n/ for it. It may help to elicit the place of the /ŋ/ at this point since clients are less likely to feel their tongue at the velum. When clients have difficulties with this sound, see if the sound exists allophonically as a result of assimilation in their language, which might help them develop a feel for how the sound is produced.

The approximants of English consist of two liquids, /ɹ, l/ and two glides, /w,j/. Of the liquids, the /l/ usually presents fewer challenges since it is such a common sound in the world's languages, but there are a few exceptions. Japanese does not have /ɹ/ or /l/ and uses a voiced alveolar lateral flap [ɺ] that is different from both, so Japanese clients may have difficulties with both English liquids. Appendix 6–3 features some minimal pairs that can be used with Japanese clients. Speakers of the Sichuan dialect of Mandarin may alternate /n/ and /l/ as mentioned above. Some clients may have difficulties with /l/ due to phonotactics, in which case they might produce it well word initially, but vocalize it word finally. Speakers of Portuguese (especially Brazilians) and Mandarin typically produce labialized or vocalized word-final /l/, so a word like *ball* might come out as [baʊ̯].

One area that usually merits attention is the dark /l/ allophone, represented in IPA as [ɫ]. In many languages, the /l/ is produced with less allophonic variation than in our language. In English, the /l/ in a word like *light* is different than the [ɫ] in *call*. We usually make the /l/ at the beginning of a word with the tongue at the alveolar ridge or even interdentally, but when it comes at the end of a syllable there is secondary velarization, with the body of the tongue further back. There is a great deal of variation among speakers and dialects, but one characteristic of American English is the frequent tendency to use the [ɫ]. Native speakers are not consciously aware of these differences and they are unlikely to affect ineligibility in any way, but clinicians can help their clients sound more natural by shaping these final /l/ sounds.

The American /ɹ/ sound is generally more challenging because clients will not have the same tactile cues they have for the /l/. Unlike the /l/, for which they should be able to feel their tongue touch at the alveolar ridge and can sing out some syllables to feel the lateral nature of the sound, the /ɹ/ is a complex non-visual sound that is rarely in the phonemic inventories of clients' native languages. This phoneme is probably not worth a significant investment of time during an overview of the consonants, but clinicians can give clients some advice about using their ears to shape their production of the /ɹ/ sound.

The final two approximants are the glides /w,j/. The /w/ is less common in other languages, and many clients will substitute a /v/ for it. Since it is primarily a labial sound (with secondary velar articulation), it is visual, and clients can practice with a mirror. It is also unlikely that the substitution will affect intelligibility significantly. When words are spelled with "wh," some native speakers use a voiceless labial-velar fricative, represented in the IPA as [ʍ], thus the word *when* might be pronounced [ʍɛn] and not [wɛn]. This allophone is in free variation and appears to be becoming rarer. While clinicians who use it in their own speech can practice this sound with their clients, it is probably safer to simply develop clients' awareness of it and encourage them to use the /w/. It is less likely that clients will need to work on the /j/ phoneme, but since it is a semivowel, the best way to elicit it is to have clients extend the /i/ vowel as far as possible and then shape it into a /j/. It represents the only palatal phoneme in English.

# Problematic Phonemes

## Typical Targets

Since intelligibility is crucial to communicative success, clinicians usually focus on phonemes over allophones because they have the greatest impact on clients' ability to get their message across accurately. In theory, a client may need training to produce accurate versions of virtually any consonant of English, but for all practical purposes, the actual set is usually limited. It is often best to start with consonants since those are the most concrete phonemes and SLPs will be coming at them from a position of strength due to their training. Clinicians can establish trust by attaining good results up front with consonants and then branching out to vowels and suprasegmentals. If an assessment has been done, the clinician should have an idea about which consonants to target, but a minimal pairs diagnostic, as exemplified by Appendix 6–4, can be used if needed. The most common consonant phoneme targets in accent modification are /ɹ,θ,ð,ʤ,w,h/, and another set, /ŋ,v,ʧ,ʒ,l,ʃ,z,f,j/, can be considered the next tier. This is not a science-based or a recommended order, but just a reflection of tendencies. Clinicians always need to choose targets carefully considering the client's L1 phonology, the impact on intelligibility and naturalness, stimulability, ease, and many other variables. The overarching principles involved in training clients on segmentals were outlined in Chapter 4. Since minimal pairs are such a common technique for working on consonants, Appendix 6–5 features numerous examples. It is always recommended that clients develop a keen awareness of minimal pairs that involve sounds that are difficult for them, and they should be encouraged to come up with their own lists.

One thing that may jump out immediately when looking at the list of typical targets is the absence of stops, which are usually addressed only in terms of their allophonic variations in English. The stops are common in the world's languages, with some notable exceptions such as the lack of /p/ in Arabic. Most of the difficulties clients have with these consonants relate to aspiration or release. The list also has some overlap with targets that are common when working with children. Of the "late eight," only the /s/ is missing. The voiceless sounds are also in the minority, since 10 of the 15 sounds from the two groups of phonemes that cause difficulty for clients are voiced.

## American /ɹ/

As outlined above, the American /ɹ/ presents many challenges for clients and clinicians alike, and a detailed review of its production and shaping are beyond the scope of this book. The good news is that there are many books available on this subject, and many SLPs have websites and tutorials dedicated to this sound. The 2nd edition of Secord and Secord's *Eliciting Sounds* (2007) dedicates an entire chapter to "/r/ and /ɚ/: From Science to Practice," which provides a detail on the different ways Americans produce this sound. One of the difficulties when working with this sound is that there are two major ways to produce it: retroflex and "bunched," but Secord points out that there is quite a bit of variation involved in both productions. Another difficulty is the fact that visual cues are not of much use; to help clients with the /θ, ð/ a mirror will sometimes do the trick, but for the /ɹ/, you might need an fMRI! The /ɹ/ is a high-frequency sound in English, ranking 3rd of the consonants and 5th overall (Edwards, 1992), but it is difficult to categorize since it can be said to function as both a consonant sound, and postvocalically as a vowel sound, and this ranking probably underestimates the outsized role the rhotic vowels play in producing natural American speech.

Clients may begin accent modification with an approximation of an American /ɹ/, or typically, they will use a trill /r/. Some clients may also use the alveolar tap /ɾ/, a uvular trill /ʀ/, or a voiced uvular fricative /ʁ/, and clinicians will need to decide the overall impact on intelligibility. Clients who substitute an /r/ will usually be understood well since native speakers of English are quite familiar with that feature of many non-native accents, and /r/ is not in our inventory. While in some cases, an inaccurate /ɹ/ or a substitution of a non-English phoneme affects intelligibility, it is bound to affect naturalness, as native speakers will notice it every time. It is a common sound, and more importantly, inaccurate productions will have a large impact on vowel sounds because of the rhoticity of American English.

Most clients who produce an inaccurate /ɹ/ or use a substitution do not have issues related to perception, so training can focus entirely on production. They typically have a phoneme similar to an /l/, so when they hear an English /l/, it can go right in that slot, and when they hear an English /ɹ/ they can put it in the slot where they have some type of trill or approximant. However, Japanese clients will often have difficulties with perception and production. When SLPs work with children, they expect perception to precede production, but Japanese speakers do not always follow that pattern. When Japanese speakers hear /ɹ, l/ they are not able to sort them into two categories since both of them map onto their /l/. Surprisingly, they are often able to create approximations of the expected sounds if they know which one to produce. In other words, a Japanese speaker will often be able to produce distinct versions of /ɹ, l/, but still identify them at a chance rate when listening. Clinicians should recognize that in this case, perception may not actually help the client produce the sounds better, even though it is obviously important for listening comprehension. Nevertheless, minimal pairs with /ɹ, l/ are certainly an obvious approach to target perception and production in this population. For other clients, minimal pairs may be less effective since they probably produce a non-ambient phoneme in English, and in this case, clinicians can use word lists that feature the /ɹ/ in various positions. Clients can also work with phrases or texts that are /ɹ/-heavy, and because of its frequency, it should be easy to focus on productions during spontaneous speech activities of any kind.

## The *th* /θ, ð/

The next two consonants that are commonly targeted are the "th" sounds /θ, ð/, and it is hard to imagine a pronunciation text in the ESL market that does not address them. Despite their status as one of the top targets, there is debate about whether they are appropriate choices since they are often considered to have low functional load. The sounds themselves are relatively rare, and non-native speakers may even feel strange about sticking their tongues out during speech if their language uses that gesture exclusively paralinguistically to express anger or some other emotion. The most common substitutions are /t/ or /s/ for /θ/, and /d/ or /z/ for /ð/. In almost every case, speakers of a particular language make the same substitution , so while a speaker from the Netherlands might use a /d/, someone from France will substitute /z/. This book makes the case that these sounds deserve their high rank as goals for accent modification.

There is both good news and bad news when it comes to the interdental fricatives and non-native speakers. Starting with the bad news for clients, while they are generally absent in the inventories of most of the world's languages, they are not rare phonemes in English. The /ð/is ranked ninth in frequency among the consonant sounds of English and /θ/ comes in toward the bottom, at 20th out of 24 (Edwards, 1992). This may understate their overall importance somewhat, since they occur in such high-frequency words as *the*, *that*, and *with*, which are all in the top 15 most common words of English, with the word *the* occupying the number one slot. On the other hand, the good news is that these sounds have the benefit of being highly visual, so both clinicians and clients can use visual feedback (with a mirror or video) to shape their production. Native speakers do not always produce this sound with the tongue completely through the teeth, but non-native speakers should always be encouraged to produce it this way until they can learn to be more flexible in terms of natural sounding allophones. Another bit of good news is that orthographically, these sounds are spelled with "th" 100% of the time, and the converse is generally true—if a word is spelled with "th," there are only a few exceptions (such as *Thomas*) where neither phoneme is produced. One more piece of bad news is that there is no easy way to distinguish whether "th" will be produced as /θ/ or /ð/. To put yourself in the non-native speaker's position, imagine that you have to learn a language that uses the "v" letter to represent both /f/ and /v/, and you just have to memorize which one to produce each time you learn the word. Fortunately, there are some clues that might help clients, such as the fact that /ð/ rarely occurs word finally.

In addressing the functional load question, the good news is that there are really no common minimal pairs to worry about that contrast these two sounds themselves. We can find pairs, such as *either/ether*, but there is little chance that substituting these words would ever cause misunderstanding. Unfortunately, there also is a bit of bad news in the fact that there are indeed minimal pairs contrasting both phonemes with their likely substitutions, such as *thought/taught*, *think/sink*, *then/den*, or *clothing/closing*. Those arguing against work on these targets may downplay the impact of these pairs on intelligibility, claiming that "I thank you" produced as "I sank you" will be understood, and they are probably right, but there is little doubt that it will affect naturalness and may even lead to embarrassment for the speaker. In keeping with the clear and natural approach, this phoneme is likely to be of significant benefit in helping clients convey their message without their listeners focusing on how they are saying it. Another argument used to minimize the functional load of these sounds is that they are often absent from other varieties of English, which is true. English speakers of regional dialects in Ireland, Southern England, and New York city, as well as speakers of social dialects, such as African American English, produce these fricatives as dental stops or use other substitutions. The counter-argument would be that the sounds are used in most dialects of American English, and that non-native speakers may be judged differently than speakers of regional dialects. On a final note, to reiterate a point from above, the /θ, ð/ phonemes are visual, and clinicians should be able to train clients in how to produce these sounds in virtually every case even if generalization takes longer. By focusing on these sounds, especially at the beginning of training, clients can get some early success in articulatory accuracy that is certain to promote clearer and more natural speech once generalization begins.

Clinicians can use combinations of the approaches described above, and certainly, minimal pairs represent one option, although there is usually not much point in working with the limited set of minimal pairs that contrast the two sounds themselves. Tongue twisters, as well as phrases and texts rich in "th," are also good options, and the frequency of these sounds in everyday speech means that there should be plenty of opportunity to monitor generalization when clients speak spontaneously. Appendix 6–6 features some minimal pairs for "th" as well as a text to help clients focus on its pronunciation.

## The Post-Alveolar Affricates /tʃ, dʒ/

These phonemes are both produced by stopping the airflow initially and then releasing into a continuant, represented by the fricative symbol in the IPA character. They are, however, not completely identical to a stop plus fricative, and native speakers perceive them as one sound. Although these two are paired together here, the marked phoneme /dʒ/ usually represents more of a challenge for clients due to its voicing, and it is common for some clients to substitute the /tʃ/ for the /dʒ/ if their language has the former and not the latter. In languages such as Spanish, /tʃ/ may be an allophone of /ʃ/, depending on the dialect, so Spanish speakers might deaffricate. Production can also be very context dependent, so in languages that have final consonant devoicing, the /dʒ/ in final position can be more challenging. Some languages, such as Korean, typically add a vowel after these final consonants, so *judge* might be produced as something like [dʒʌdʒɪ]. The sounds themselves are both low frequency, with /dʒ, tʃ/ coming in at the 22nd and 23rd out of the 24 most common consonants sounds, respectively (Edwards, 1992), which should certainly be considered when deciding whether to select them as targets. If clients have the unvoiced affricate in their phonetic inventory, but not its counterpart, they can practice voicing contrasting the sounds in medial or initial position. Remember that when contrasting them word finally, the most salient difference is in the length of the vowel, which is longer before the voiced phoneme. Clients should focus on this length distinction if they are having difficulty producing the voiced version in final position. Naturally, if the client is deaffricating, then the appropriate contrast would be the resulting fricative.

## The Remaining Approximants, /w, j, l/, and the Glottal Fricative /h/

All four English approximants are common accent modification targets, depending on the client's L1. The /l/ generally presents the least challenge, with the exceptions of some dialects of Mandarin, and the Japanese /l, ɹ/ issue, as mentioned above. The main concern is usually allophonic, that is, the use of dark /ɫ/. The /j/ is also usually not a significant problem in and of itself, since it can be elicited fairly easily from the /i/ vowel sound, but it may be used as a substitution for another phoneme, such as the /dʒ/, or it might be epenthetically inserted before vowels, as when the word *ears* is produced as *years*. The remaining two (/w, h/) present more difficulty for speakers of certain languages, and many languages lack one or both of them. In languages that don't have the /w/, the /v/ is often substituted if the L1 has the /v/ phoneme. The visual nature of the /w/ (apart from the secondary velar articulation) means that visual feedback can be used to ensure that the client's teeth do not touch the lips. The /w/ is a semivowel that can be shaped from the /u/, so for example, in guiding clients to produce the word *would*, the clinician can start with something like [uʊd] and then merge and shape the initial sounds. Since this sound is generally easier to elicit, the main difficulty comes with generalization. Lastly, the /h/ represents a significant challenge for speakers of languages that have neither this sound itself, nor a suitable substitute such as a voiceless velar fricative /x/ or a voiceless palatal fricative /ç/. For example, native Russian- and Spanish-speaking clients do not have the /h/ in their inventories, but by substituting the /x/ they are able to produce distinct versions of *hate* and *ate* and will have less chance of reduced intelligibility than L1 speakers who do not have /h/ or any substitutions in their phonemic inventory such as speakers of French, who often struggle and need to focus carefully in order to produce the /h/. The /h/ is somewhat of an elusive sound, and phoneticians do not agree on the best way to categorize it. The IPA lists it as a fricative, but Ladefoged (2004) points out that there is virtually no friction in the glottis when it is produced, so it can be difficult to describe. Clinicians can work with clients to ensure that the sound is produced much more lightly than fricatives produced further along the vocal tract.

# Allophones

## Natural Speech

Much of what distinguishes accents and dialects at the segmental level relates to allophonic variation. In some cases, these variations may be barely perceptible, as is the case with voice onset time, where variance measured in milliseconds can be the difference between a native or non-native production. In other cases, the distinction is very noticeable; the use of the alveolar tap is easily recognized as a feature of American English as opposed to British English. When accent modification is focused entirely on producing intelligible speech, these variations may be overlooked, but they play a large role in helping clients sound more natural. The alveolar tap serves as a perfect example. If a non-native speaker pronounces the word *water* as /watɚ/ as opposed to /waɾɚ/, there is little likelihood of misunderstanding, especially since the use of a /t/ is common in many dialects of English. If we are aiming strictly for intelligibility, we could even make the case that using a /t/ is preferred here. However, this overlooks the fact that native speakers will notice this difference each time it occurs and will spend time thinking about the non-native speaker's pronunciation. To balance clear and natural speech, the alveolar tap should be high on the list of targets.

Before looking at which allophones are the most important for accent modification training, let's review how allophones work and their distribution patterns. Allophones differ from phonemes in the sense that they do not change the meaning of a word. While phonemes are considered to be in contrastive distribution because replacing one with another creates a word with a different meaning, allophones can be in either free variation or complementary variation. If they are in free variation, then speakers have a choice in whether to use them or not. An example of an allophone in free variation is the final /t/ in a word like *cat* since speakers can release it or produce it with no audible release and the meaning of the word does not change. Native speakers may have limited awareness of when they or others are actually producing different allophones in free variation, and the decision to produce one allophone or another is rarely made at the conscious level. In most cases, a particular allophone may be preferred, but if another allophone in free variation is used, it may not even be noticed. In contrast, speakers have no choice but to produce allophones that are in complementary distribution, and the allophone is determined entirely by context. With allophones in complementary distribution, listeners will notice immediately if a different allophone is produced.

## The Alveolar Tap

The alveolar tap, symbolized in the IPA as /ɾ/, is one of the most salient features of American English (as well as some other English dialects such as Canadian English and Australian English), but many non-natives speakers are hesitant to use it and have little understanding of the rules governing it. In some cases, clients come to the United States after learning English in countries where British English is the most common form used in classrooms and textbooks, as is often the cases in countries of the European Union, and the tap may have been discouraged. Learners exposed to American English notice the difference very quickly, but since they receive little instruction regarding this allophone, they may feel safer producing a /t/. If they turn to native speakers for help, they are unlikely to receive useful guidance since most native speakers have a poor understanding of how it functions and would have difficulty explaining it. Clinicians should encourage clients to master the tap if they are planning to communicate with speakers of American English since it will help their listeners focus on what they are saying as opposed to how they are saying it. The tap in a word such as *water* is so universal in American English, that it is safe to say that the /t/ is used in that word only in imitation of another dialect, as a form of mockery, to project in extremely loud environments, or when conversing with speakers who have limited English proficiency.

Clients often feel empowered when the mysteries of the tap are revealed to them, and they are typically surprised that the rules are fairly regular. Most clients who communicate in American English will use the tap in some but not all of the normal contexts, and it is common for clients to use it in everyday words such as *water* while avoiding it in words they say less often such as *native*. Because it will not result in miscommunication, it is unlikely that native speakers will correct them, and these habits will easily become ingrained. The alveolar tap has a peculiar status in American English; technically it is in complementary distribution because ears would certainly perk up if a native speaker pronounced the word *potato* as /pəteɪtoʊ/, but native speakers will occasionally use it when they are overenunciating, and they are certainly more aware of the control they have over it than they are of the amount of aspiration they might put on an initial /t/. Some Americans seem to feel that there is something wrong with the tap allophone, but it is difficult to identify the reasons for this mild stigmatization. Although it's important to determine which variety of English clients aspire to speak, clients will sound more natural in American English if they use the tap regularly.

Clinicians should probe clients' awareness of the tap to see if they understand the nature of the sound and when to produce it. One way of doing this is to take a word that features both a /t/ and /ɾ/ and then pronounce it with two /t/ sounds, two /ɾ/ sounds and then the typical American English way, with one of each, and see if clients can determine which one sounds most natural in American English. For example, you can pronounce *potato* as [pəteɪtoʊ], [pəɾeɪɾoʊ], and [pəteɪɾoʊ] in any order to see if clients are aware of which version is the most common. When asked to describe the /ɾ/, clients will usually say that it sounds "like a d," and clinicians should agree, and explain the speed element, and possibly compare a word with a stop /d/ and a tap. On a side note, some non-native speakers (such as Spanish speakers) may say that the tap is like an "r" because in these languages, the tap does serve as an "r," or one type of "r." For example, the Spanish word *caro* (meaning expensive, or dear) is pronounced /kaɾo/ and has the minimal pair *carro* /karo/, which means "car." When clients respond this way, it is a great opportunity to discuss the "r" along with the tap, and often the client will gain a much better grasp of the /ɾ/. It is helpful to use the term *tap* or *flap* and to introduce the IPA symbol to help clients develop an awareness of its importance, but some clinicians just call it a "fast d" or just a "d." In phonetics the term *tap* seems to be preferred to *flap* for this sound in English, but the terms are often used interchangeably.

The rules for the tap can be explained quickly to clients, and then the focus should be on practicing and watching for generalization. When /t/ or /d/ occur between vowels they become the alveolar tap /ɾ/ unless the second vowel is in a stressed syllable. The word *Italy* is produced with a tap [ɪɾəli] because the /t/ is between two vowels and the stress is on the first syllable. In the word *Italian*, there is no tap and the word is pronounced with a /t/ because the second syllable is stressed. Another way of thinking of this is that the tap cannot lead into a stressed syllable. Clients should note that initial /t/ and final /t/ are never taps. Although technically the /d/ becomes a flap under the same circumstances, it is less important to point this out to students and it might be an unnecessary distraction, since there is a much smaller difference between /t/ and /ɾ/ than /d/ and /ɾ/. It may also help to point out that words with the tap sound different from their British English counter-parts. The words *writer* and *rider* will sound much more similar in American English than in British English: [ɹaɪɾɚ] and [ɹaɪːɾɚ] versus [ɹaɪtə] and [ɹaɪːdə]. For advanced speakers, it may be worth pointing out that some native speakers of American English pronounce *writer* with a shorter vowel than *rider* due to the underlying /t/ phoneme, while for other native speakers, the words are homophones. Clinicians can also point out to their more advanced clients that while /t/ is virtually always pronounced as a tap when the syllable before the /t/ is stressed, at times some speakers pronounce the /t/ as a /t/ intervocalically between two unstressed syllables in longer words. In other words, it would be unusual for an American English speaker to pronounce either /t/ in the word *automatic* as a /t/; compare [ˌɑtəˈmætɪk] to [ˌɑɾəˈmæɾɪk]. Depending on dialect, idiolect, and context, the word *automaticity* might be pronounced with either a tap or a /t/ at the end because it is between two unstressed vowels, as in [ˌɑɾəmæˈtɪsɪti] versus [ˌɑɾəmæˈtɪsɪɾi]. While there is no harm in working on the tap with speakers of any level of English proficiency, these more advanced rules may not be appropriate for beginners and intermediate-level clients, especially if clients are struggling with stress in general.

Once clients have developed some awareness of what the tap is and the rules that govern it, they can work on identifying words containing taps. Clinicians can use lists of words featuring some /t/ and some /ɾ/ sounds so clients can see words such as *attack*, *attic, automatic, attention* and then either identify the taps while looking at them or read them aloud accurately. As an additional contrast, include some words that are spelled with a "t" but are pronounced with a /ʧ/, like *natural*. After clients can produce the tap in structured practice activities, clinicians should spend a considerable amount of time monitoring clients' spontaneous speech for carryover.

## The Nasal Tap

A logical pivot from the alveolar tap is to begin to develop clients' awareness of the nasal tap, symbolized in the IPA by [ɾ̃]. This allophone occurs when "nt" in English is between vowels, and where the second vowel is an unstressed syllable. For example, American English speakers will produce the word *winter* as either [wɪntɚ] or [wɪɾ̃ɚ]. By substituting the nasal tap for "nt," homophones can occur that would not exist in other varieties of English; in this case *winter* produced as [wɪɾ̃ɚ] is indistinguishable from the word *winner*. This allophone is in free variation, so it is important to point out to clients that they are free to choose which version they prefer. Native speakers tend to use the nasal tap more frequently than "nt," but this depends on context, and it is generally less common in careful speech. One way of developing awareness of relative frequency is to give clients a list of two or three common words such as *center, twenty,* or even *internet* and ask them to note how they hear native speakers pronounce them spontaneously during any given week. They should be cautioned that asking native speakers directly how to pronounce any of these words will likely result in /nt/ and not the nasal tap since natives tend to produce citation forms in these situations. This type of assignment helps clients concentrate on the speech stream around them. They typically report back that the nasal tap is much more common than "nt." Another way of looking at this variation is to treat it as elision of the /t/, and there is nothing wrong with that approach if it makes more sense during training. By identifying it as a nasal tap, clients can apply the same basic rules that they have learned for the alveolar tap, provided that they understand that this allophone is in free and not complementary distribution.

Clients can practice identifying words that contain the nasal tap as they did with the alveolar tap, but it is essential to remind them that there are no right or wrong answers here. It may be beneficial to see if clients can identify words with the nasal tap that may be less obvious to them. For example, most clients learn quickly that Americans tend to pronounce *twenty* as [twɛɾ̃i], but they may not realize that *wanted* is usually [wɑɾ̃ɪd]. In addition, when monitoring clients' spontaneous speech production, clinicians can remind them of the possibility of using this allophone, but in comparison to the alveolar tap, the priority of pointing this out should be much lower because both options are possible.

## Unreleased Stops

Another common allophonic variation is to produce final stop consonants with no audible release, symbolized by the IPA [ ̚ ] diacritic. For example, the word *hit* is usually produced as [hɪt̚] and the final stop is not released. To demonstrate this to clients, a word like *lap* is helpful because when the final /p/ is not released, clinicians can demonstrate that the lips are still closed when the word ends. In contrast to many of the allophonic variations that affect only the voiceless stops, this applies to the voiced stops as well.

Many clients have L1s that do not allow production of final stops in this manner, so they will be fighting against a lifelong habit. If they have received pronunciation instruction aimed squarely at intelligibility, it is unlikely that this was discussed. Structured practice with words ending in stops can make this more automatic for clients, and a mirror may come in handy so that the client can monitor the position of the articulators at the end of the word. Once again, it is important to develop clients' awareness of how common this is in typical American English speech. As a homework assignment, clinicians can ask clients to listen to native speakers throughout the week and try to estimate the approximate ratio of released and unreleased stops. It may be easier for them to focus on the released versions, since those are generally rarer, and in doing so, clients will come to realize that no audible release is the norm.

In a similar vein, clients can be taught that stops are generally unreleased when they precede other consonants, so the /p/ in the word *captain* is held and then the /t/ is released. This allophonic variation might be best addressed in more detail when working with linking and some of the other features of connected speech.

## The Glottal Stop

This allophone is usually addressed by clinicians only if it is being incorrectly substituted, as in the case of clients who might use it at word boundaries instead of linking smoothly, but it is a good idea to give clients some awareness of its allophonic role in English. We tend to think of it as just the sound we make when we are saying "uh oh," but in reality, it is used much more commonly than that, albeit never phonemically. When words or phrases begin with a vowel, we tend to use an initial glottal stop instead of easing into the vowel, and in most cases clients will either do this spontaneously already, or if not, native speakers may not even notice. It is often used lightly as a link between certain vowels, as in the break between the words *saw* and *Alex* in "I saw Alex." Some native speakers use it to link the word *the* to another word starting with a vowel as in "the act" as [ðəʔækt], although others prefer a front vowel and glide [ðiʲækt]. Perhaps, the most practical use for clients is in simplifying sequences of consonants, as in a word like *atmosphere*, which is normally produced as [æʔməsfɪɚ], or across word boundaries, such as *fat chance*. which could come out as [fæʔʧænts].

## Syllabic /n/

Many clients have difficulty producing accurate versions of words such as *written* because they pronounce a /t/ and use two vowels, so while the non-native speaker's version of the word *written* would sound like [ɹɪtɛn̩], the native version is generally something like [ɹɪʔn̩]. The non-native speakers' version will be highly intelligible, but it will diverge significantly from the natural model produced by native speakers. It is easiest to tackle the extra vowel and have the client replace it with the syllabic /n/ before looking at the glottal stop in place of the /t/. Clinicians can point out the types of words in which this process is likely to occur, namely in words that feature /t/ before /n/ in final unstressed syllables. Examples are words such as *Latin*, *certain*, and *cotton*. Once clients have noted that there is now vowel between the /t/ and the /n/, clinicians can have them produce the /n/ sound in isolation, making sure that there is no vowel preceding or following it. Clients should practice with words that end in /s/ plus [n̩] such as *listen* and *fasten* because those are generally easier to produce natural than words such as *cotton* or *certain*. The more difficult task is for clients to replace the /t/ with a glottal stop, since they usually have produced these types of words exclusively with a /t/, and they have to invest some effort in unlearning this. As with all allophones, clients should not be discouraged if they struggle to produce accurate versions, and clinicians can point out that they will not be in danger of being misunderstood if they produce these words with a /t/.

## Nasal Plosion

The next logical allophonic variation is the nasal plosion that occurs in words with a final unstressed /d/ + /n/ sequence, such as the words *sudden* and *widen*. Clients tend to produce these types of words with full vowels, so *sudden* may come out as [sʌdɛn] as opposed to the more typical native version [sʌdn̩]. Clients can practice placing their tongues at the alveolar ridge to produce the /d/ and then dropping their velum to produce the nasal. Appendix 6–7 features examples of prompts to target taps, syllabic /n/, and nasal plosion.

## References

Dryer, M. S., & Haspelmath, M. (eds.) (2013). *The World Atlas of Language Structures Online*. Leipzig: Max Planck Institute for Evolutionary Anthropology. (Available online at http://wals.info, Retrieved on 2018-12-09.)

Edwards, H. T. (1992). *Applied phonetics: Instructor's Manual*. San Diego, CA: Singular Publishing Group.

International Phonetic Association (2014). *Handbook of the International Phonetic Association: A guide to the use of the International Phonetic Alphabet*. Cambridge, UK: Cambridge University Press.

Ladefoged, P. (2004). *A course in phonetics*. Boston, MA: Thomson Wadsworth.

Ladefoged, P. (2005). *Vowels and consonants: An introduction to the sounds of languages*. Malden, MA: Wiley-Blackwell.

Pereltsvaig, A. *Sounds and sound systems around the world: An (sic) brief overview*. Retrieved from: https://www.languagesoftheworld.info/linguistic-typology/sounds-sound-systems-around-world-brief-overview.html

Secord, W., (2007). *Eliciting sounds: Techniques and strategies for clinicians*. Clifton Park, NY: Thomson Delmar Learning.

# 6-1

# Thinking About Consonants

A. What are some examples of consonants? How can you define *consonant*?

B. Close your eyes and make the following sounds. As you do so, think about which parts of your mouth are used to stop the air.

/p/ as in the first and last sound of *pop*
/t/ as in the first and last sound in *tight*
/k/ as in the first and last sounds in *cook*

C. Now try these continuous sounds. Where are they made?

/f/ as in the first sound in *fit*
/θ/ as in the first sound in *thin*
/s/ as in the first sound in *see*
/ʃ/ as in the first sound in *she*

D. Which of the following beginning sounds can you make continuously?

**t**op, **sh**op, **ch**op

E. Say the following words and keep saying the final sound as long as you can.

ram          ran         rang

What do they have in common? What makes them different?

F. Say the words *light* and *right* and stretch out the first sounds. What is the difference in how you make them?

G. Say the following words. How do you make the first sound in each one?

hay         way         yay

# 6-2

# Minimal Pairs: Voicing

## Final Continuants

|   | Unvoiced | Voiced | Contrast |
|---|----------|--------|----------|
| 1 | price | prize | /s/ vs. /z/ |
| 2 | loose | lose | |
| 3 | place | plays | |
| 4 | use (noun) | use (verb) | |
| 5 | leaf | leave | /f/ vs. /v/ |
| 6 | half | have | |
| 7 | belief | believe | |
| 8 | etch | edge | /tʃ/ vs. /dʒ/ |
| 9 | "h" | age | |
| 10 | search | surge | |

## Final Stops

|   | Unvoiced | Voiced | Contrast |
|---|----------|--------|----------|
| 1 | lap | lab | /p/ vs. /b/ |
| 2 | rip | rib | |
| 3 | mop | mob | |
| 4 | back | bag | /k/ vs. /g/ |
| 5 | lake | leg | |

| 6 | dock | dog | |
|---|------|-----|---|
| 7 | bat | bad | /t/ vs. /d/ |
| 8 | wet | wed | |
| 9 | mate | made | |

## Initial Stops

| | Unvoiced | Voiced | Contrast |
|---|----------|--------|----------|
| 1 | pad | bad | /p/ vs. /b/ |
| 2 | pig | big | |
| 3 | palm | bomb | |
| 4 | come | gum | /k/ vs. /g/ |
| 5 | came | game | |
| 6 | cut | gut | |
| 7 | time | dime | /t/ vs. /d/ |
| 8 | tile | dial | |
| 9 | tore | door | |

# 6-3

# Worksheet: /r/ and /l/ Minimal Pairs

|    | A. /r/  | B. /l/  |
|----|---------|---------|
| 1  | rock    | lock    |
| 2  | race    | lace    |
| 3  | correct | collect |
| 4  | pirate  | pilot   |
| 5  | fry     | fly     |
| 6  | crown   | clown   |
| 7  | car     | call    |
| 8  | bore    | bowl    |
| 9  | rather  | lather  |
| 10 | rip     | lip     |
| 11 | pier    | peel    |
| 12 | rate    | late    |
| 13 | ray     | lay     |
| 14 | poor    | pole    |
| 15 | rot     | lot     |

## /r/ and /l/ Minimal Pairs in Sentences

|    | A. /r/ | B. /l/ |
|----|--------|--------|
| 1  | This really feels right. | This really feels light. |
| 2  | Did you bring the surprise? | Did you bring the supplies? |
| 3  | I think we took the wrong road. | I think we took the long road. |
| 4  | The child wanted to see the crown. | The child wanted to see the clown. |
| 5  | Don't stand in the rain. | Don't stand in the lane. |
| 6  | Can we pay that rate? | Can we pay that late? |
| 7  | He had a red soldier. | He had a lead soldier. |
| 8  | Did you see the pirate? | Did you see the pilot? |
| 9  | He rocked the car. | He locked the car. |
| 10 | She doesn't fry very often. | She doesn't fly very often. |
| 11 | He refused to correct it. | He refused to collect it. |
| 12 | That guy's really rude. | That guy's really lewd. |
| 13 | Give me a car. | Give me a call. |
| 14 | He fell in the batter. | He fell in the battle. |

# 6-4

# Sample Worksheet Minimal Pairs Diagnostic: Consonants

| # | A | B | Contrast |
|---|---|---|---|
| 1 | ban | van | /b/ vs. /v/ |
| 2 | robe | rove | |
| 3 | thick | sick | /θ/ vs. /s/ |
| 4 | math | mass | |
| 5 | vent | went | /v/ vs. /w/ |
| 6 | rover | rower | |
| 7 | breathe | breeze | /ð/ vs. /z/ |
| 8 | then | Zen | |
| 9 | jealous | zealous | /dʒ/ vs. /z/ |
| 10 | fudge | fuzz | |
| 11 | yell | gel | /j/ vs. /dʒ/ |
| 12 | weighing | waging | |
| 13 | night | light | /n/ vs. /l/ |
| 14 | ten | tell | |
| 15 | pan | fan | /p/ vs. /f/ |

| 16 | cheap | chief | |
|----|-------|-------|---|
| 17 | gone | gong | /n/ vs. /ŋ/ |
| 18 | sinner | singer | |
| 19 | thank | tank | /θ/ vs. /t/ |
| 20 | myth | mitt | |
| 21 | see | she | /s/ vs. /ʃ/ |
| 22 | class | clash | |
| 23 | those | doze | /ð/ vs. /z/ |
| 24 | bathe | bays | |
| 25 | choke | joke | /tʃ/ vs. /dʒ/ |
| 26 | batch | badge | |
| 27 | etching | edging | |
| 28 | rice | lice | /r/ vs. /l/ |
| 29 | fire | file | |
| 30 | correct | collect | |
| 31 | bash | badge | /ʃ/ vs. /dʒ/ |
| 32 | shames | James | |
| 33 | slushy | sludgy | |
| 34 | wish | witch | /ʃ/ vs. /tʃ/ |
| 35 | share | chair | |
| 36 | washing | watching | |

# 6-5

# Supplemental Consonant Minimal Pairs

1. /b/ /v/

|   | A. /b/ | B. /v/ |
|---|--------|--------|
| 1 | ban | van |
| 2 | bee | v |
| 3 | berry | very |
| 4 | bowel | vowel |
| 5 | bent | vent |
| 6 | bicker | vicar |
| 7 | curb | curve |
| 8 | bow | vow |

2. /f/ /p/

|   | A. /f/ | B. /p/ |
|---|--------|--------|
| 1 | fit | pit |
| 2 | laugh | lap |
| 3 | fat | pat |
| 4 | suffer | supper |
| 5 | cough | cop |

| 6 | coffee | copy |
|---|--------|------|
| 7 | fine   | pine |
| 8 | cuff   | cup  |

## 3. /f/ /v/

|   | A. /f/ | B. /v/  |
|---|--------|---------|
| 1 | fan    | van     |
| 2 | fine   | vine    |
| 3 | thief  | thieve  |
| 4 | belief | believe |
| 5 | half   | have    |
| 6 | fairy  | very    |
| 7 | infest | invest  |
| 8 | fat    | vat     |

## 4. /θ/ /ð/

|   | A. /θ/ | B. /ð/  |
|---|--------|---------|
| 1 | mouth  | mouthe  |
| 2 | thigh  | thy     |
| 3 | teeth  | teethe  |
| 4 | ether  | either  |

## 5. /s/ /ʃ/

|   | A. /s/ | B. /ʃ/  |
|---|--------|---------|
| 1 | see    | she     |
| 2 | Sue    | shoe    |
| 3 | seed   | She'd   |
| 4 | seep   | sheep   |
| 5 | sip    | ship    |
| 6 | plus   | plush   |
| 7 | gas    | gash    |
| 8 | crass  | crash   |

6. /ʃ/ /ʧ/

|   | A. /ʃ/ | B. /tʃ/ |
|---|--------|---------|
| 1 | wish | witch |
| 2 | wash | watch |
| 3 | ship | chip |
| 4 | share | chair |
| 5 | washer | watcher |
| 6 | wishing | witching |
| 7 | washed | watched |
| 8 | mush | mutch |

7. /ʃ/ /ʤ/

|   | A. /ʃ/ | B. /dʒ/ |
|---|--------|---------|
| 1 | shade | jade |
| 2 | slush | sludge |
| 3 | bash | badge |
| 4 | Shelly | jelly |
| 5 | basher | badger |
| 6 | sham | jam |
| 7 | sheep | jeep |
| 8 | shear | jeer |

8. /n/ /l/

|   | A. /n/ | B. /l/ |
|---|--------|--------|
| 1 | nine | line |
| 2 | bone | bowl |
| 3 | nap | lap |
| 4 | noose | loose |
| 5 | not | lot |
| 6 | miner | miler |
| 7 | mean | meal |
| 8 | nick | lick |

9. /v/ /w/

|   | A. /v/ | B. /w/ |
|---|--------|--------|
| 1 | very | wary |
| 2 | viper | wiper |
| 3 | verse | worse |
| 4 | vending | wending |
| 5 | vine | wine |
| 6 | vile | while |
| 7 | vent | went |
| 8 | rover | rower |

10. /tʃ/ /dʒ/

|   | A. /tʃ/ | B. /dʒ/ |
|---|---------|---------|
| 1 | cheap | jeep |
| 2 | choke | joke |
| 3 | rich | ridge |
| 4 | chunk | junk |
| 5 | match | Madge |
| 6 | etch | edge |
| 7 | etching | edging |
| 8 | "h" | age |

11. /j/ /dʒ/

|   | A. /j/ | B. /dʒ/ |
|---|--------|---------|
| 1 | Yale | jail |
| 2 | yell | gel |
| 3 | yet | jet |
| 4 | yak | Jack |
| 5 | yolk | joke |
| 6 | yellow | Jello |
| 7 | yacht | jot |
| 8 | year | jeer |

12. /n/ /ŋ/

|   | A. /n/ | B. /ŋ/ |
|---|--------|--------|
| 1 | gone   | gong   |
| 2 | lawn   | long   |
| 3 | pin    | ping   |
| 4 | wins   | wings  |
| 5 | run in | running |
| 6 | stun   | stung  |
| 7 | fan    | fang   |
| 8 | sinner | singer |

# 6-6

# Worksheet: "th"

Practice avoiding substitutions with the following minimal sets:

|    | A. /θ/ | B. t | C. s |
|----|--------|------|------|
| 1  | path   | pat  | pass |
| 2  | myth   | mitt | miss |
| 3  | math   | mat  | mass |
| 4  | thick  | tick | sick |
| 5  | tenth  | tent | tense |
| 6  | thank  | tank | sank |
| 7  | thought | taught | sought |
| 8  | thin   | tin  | sin  |
| 9  | faiths | fates | face |
| 10 | thigh  | tie  | sigh |

|    | A. ð | B. d | C. z |
|----|------|------|------|
| 1  | breathing | breeding | breezing |
| 2  | seethe | seed | seize |
| 3  | lathe | laid | laze |
| 4  | bathe /beɪð/ | bade | bays |
| 5  | writhe /raɪð/ | ride | rise |
| 6  | breathe /brið/ | breed | breeze |
| 7  | scythe | side | size |
| 8  | seething | seeding | seizing |
| 9  | thee /ði/ | "d" | "z" |
| 10 | then | den | Zen |

## "th" Practice Text*

There are three men on this earth whose thoughtful advice continues to guide me through each day. The first is the man who taught me that the path to happiness goes through a thick forest filled with thousands of thorny branches. He thought that there is no way to avoid the painful thorns. The only thing you can do is guide yourself through them with all the care in the world. Another man taught me that the path to wealth goes through a thick swath of jungle, where there are thousands of threats that can lead to your death. You have to stay alert until your final breath. The third man taught me that having faith is as important as breathing, and that there is nothing that means more on this earth than that. I think that these three men were the worthiest that I've ever met.

*Voiced "th" /ð/ is underlined.

# Prompts to Target Taps, Syllabic /n/, and Nasal Plosion

**Taps.** Circle any taps in the following words:

1. committee
2. butter
3. automatic
4. attempt
5. departed
6. departure
7. toasted
8. written
9. cutting
10. tutor

**Nasal Taps.** Circle any nasal taps ([ɾ̃]) in the following words:

1. Santa Fe
2. intolerant
3. cantaloupe
4. internet
5. planted
6. plantation
7. interview

8.  counter
9.  tarantula
10. container

**Syllabic /n/.** Practice saying the following words:

1.  written
2.  beaten
3.  carton
4.  cotton
5.  certain
6.  satan

**Nasal Release.** Practice saying the following words:

1.  madden
2.  widen
3.  wooden
4.  hidden

## Tap Passage

What are the features that stand out in your mind as you think about English in the United States and Canada? The way we say words such as *water* and *winter* is certain to enter into your thoughts. It isn't that easy to identify where it is in each sentence that you ought to introduce a tap, but if you make a habit of pointing it out as you hear it, you will suddenly find out that it isn't at all that hard to make it an automatic part of your speech.

# 7

# Vowels

## Introduction to Vowels

### Out of the Comfort Zone

The importance of vowels is highlighted throughout this book because of the essential role they play in the intelligibility and naturalness of our non-native-speaking clients' speech. While working on consonants is second nature to most SLPs, they typically have less experience and training in working with this other large class of segmentals. Native-speaking children typically develop a complete vowel inventory by the age of three, and the articulation tests designed to measure childhood speech acquisition target only the consonants. Most SLPs develop a basic understanding of vowels in their undergraduate phonetics classes, and then rarely, if ever, work with vowels in their entire careers. Those who work in accent modification realize quickly the crucial role vowels play. American English has about three times the average number of vowels as typical vowel inventories of the world's languages, so they are a frequent source of difficulty for non-native speakers, and it is likely that clinicians will need to devote some time and energy to developing their own awareness and skills before working on them with clients.

### Vowel Space

Some phonetics textbooks delve into vowels before addressing consonants in detail, and many SLPs working in accent modification follow a similar order with clients because they feel they may achieve the greatest gains in this area. This book advocates for a focus on the consonants first, while keeping in mind that as long as the SLP has put thought into target selection and a logical training sequence, introducing vowels first can be equally as effective. Work on vowels and suprasegmentals is often essential for increasing clients' intelligibility and naturalness, but they are often more abstract, and clients may prefer the straightforwardness of articulation work focusing on consonants since they are more concrete. Clinicians may also be more successful in building trust with clients because vowels can cause some initial frustration. If clinicians choose to begin with consonants, there is absolutely no need to exhaust all work on them before beginning work on vowels, and an approach that starts with a few consonants and then begins integrating the vowels may prove optimal for most clients.

Vowels are more nebulous than consonants, and they are difficult to define for several reasons. The IPA chart efficiently categorizes consonants by relying primarily on place, manner, and voicing distinctions, along with nasality and laterality. Although there may be minor differences between the way a consonant phoneme is produced in different languages, the basic mechanics are easier to describe. Vowels, on the other hand, refer to a range of space, and they exist along a continuum. Clients may therefore have a more difficult time conceptualizing them, and will generally rely much more on their ears than on placement cues.

Vowel phonemes represent a range within the vowel space that is perceived as a contrastive sound by native speakers. If you take any vowel in a language and then produce equidistant variations moving toward another vowel in that language, as you approach the halfway point it becomes very difficult to determine which vowel is being produced. This is much the same way that the mind perceives color variation as you move from blue to green, for example. While the two colors are easy to identify at their respective starting points, they blend together as you move cross the boundary from one shade to the other. Even the way we break up the spectrum into colors is determined by our language and culture. In Russian, there is a word for dark blue (синий) and a word for light blue (голубой), but these can only be differentiated in English by the additional adjective. Hungarian has the word *piros* for the red used to describe a tomato versus the *vörös* used to refer to the darker color of blood. These examples are to some extent analogous to the way in which languages define and perceive vowels differently, and it helps to explain some of the difficulties non-native speakers face. The English vowel space contains the /æ/ vowel, while the German language does not, so a German speaker is likely to interpret the /æ/ vowel in a word such as *bad* as /ɛ/, since that is the closest vowel in their inventory, and produce it as /bɛd/. As native speakers of English, we will also categorize vowels from other languages within our own framework. If a German introduces himself as "Jörg" /jøːɐ̯k/, a native speaker of English is likely to call him /jɝk/, or possibly /jɝg/.

Without training, speakers of any language try to fit any nonambient vowels they hear into their existing phonological framework. They can easily hear when a vowel sounds different from those of their mother tongue, but they have difficulty identifying where they belong and producing them accurately. Clients will likely need to develop categorical perception for certain vowel contrasts that cause them trouble, but it may also be important to devote some time to this issue at the very beginning of a training program. Developing more accurate perceptions can also help with confusion related to orthography, which is particularly bothersome in terms of vowels. The IPA is a useful tool with which to begin the process of developing phonemic awareness of vowels and to disassociate their spellings.

## Developing Vowel Awareness

In comparison to the IPA symbols used to represent consonants, those representing vowels are much more dependent on conventions determined by linguists for individual languages. The IPA vowel chart maps out a range of vowels based on their degree of height, backness, and rounding, and then linguists identify the symbol that fits closest to the phonemes in each target language. While this makes the symbols much more abstract, it does not mean that there is no benefit to using IPA with non-native clients. In fact, for English, there is a distinct advantage to using IPA symbols for the vowels. The poor sound to symbol correspondence of English vowel orthography is particularly frustrating for non-native speakers. As an example, the most common vowel in English is the schwa, which can be spelled in over forty different ways (Edwards, 1992). It takes little effort to identify word pairs or sets with similar vowel spellings and entirely different pronunciations. *Good* and *food* have the same *oo* spelling but are produced with two different vowels. The minimal pair *woman/women* involves a difference in the first vowel sound /ʊ/, versus /ɪ/ (neither of which appears to correspond with the letter *o*), but in their spellings, the second vowel grapheme is the one that changes.

Clinicians can use activities to practice vowel contrasts with clients without explicit reference to the IPA. Appendix 7–1 details one such activity that features nonsense sentences containing vowel-sound pairs clients often find problematic. Nevertheless, introducing IPA to non-native speakers, particularly for troublesome vowel contrasts, helps create the awareness necessary to produce the distinction. Clients should focus on the sounds of the vowels, and not their spellings, and using IPA can help achieve that goal. An SLP, therefore, may find it particularly useful to introduce a symbol such as /æ/ and then use it in materials to disassociate any spelling interference. At some point, clients should see a chart showing all of the vowel symbols of English. Most clients begin accent modification with a limited awareness of the English vowel system, and they often confuse the number of vowel symbols used in English spelling with the number of actual vowels. When asked how many vowels there are in English, they are likely to say 5, and not the 15 or more monophthongs found in most varieties of English. In other cases, they may believe that English contains many more vowels than it actually does, so by simply identifying the number of vowels sounds in our phonemic inventory, we can create a basic awareness that builds confidence.

The use of IPA symbols helps develop categorical perception and shift clients' focus from orthography to pronunciation. One useful activity to foster knowledge of the vowel system in general, and included as Appendix 7–2, is to have clients sort lists of words containing English vowels into slots by vowel phoneme. Clinicians can also administer a type of vowel diagnostic activity with a list of minimal pairs, such as Appendix 7–3, which can help highlight vowel differences to develop phonemic awareness.

## Vowel Basics

### *Shapes and Space*

This section is not designed to replace a good phonetics textbook, which should always serve as the foundation for detailed knowledge about vowels and their allophonic variations, but rather, it offers a simple review useful for explaining these concepts to non-native speakers. One way to review vowels with clients is to discuss the concepts of categorical perception and the fact that vowels exist along an infinite spectrum. The big picture for them should be that vowels are formed by changing the shape of the space in the mouth and throat. A good analogy that clients easily grasp is the idea that if several glasses are filled with water and tapped with a knife, each produces a different sound. This can create an image of how space changes sound. However, be sure to point out that vowels are not associated with particular pitches, and any vowel can be sung as any note on the scale. The idea of resonance can help clarify this point, but it is more important to instill the idea that vowels are created by changing the shape of the space that the air from the lungs passes through.

The vowel quadrilateral can also serve as a visual representation to help clients sort out the sounds of English. One way of doing this is to start with the three vowels most commonly found in the world's languages in a simplified triangle diagram, as shown in Figure 7–1.

These may be the most common vowels in the world's languages because of their wide distance in the vowel space (Ladefoged, 2005); it is rare for a client to speak a language that does not feature something close to each of these vowels.

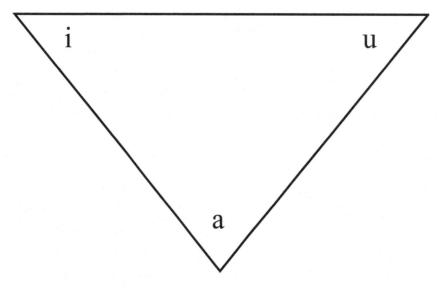

**Figure 7–1.** Typical vowel triangle.

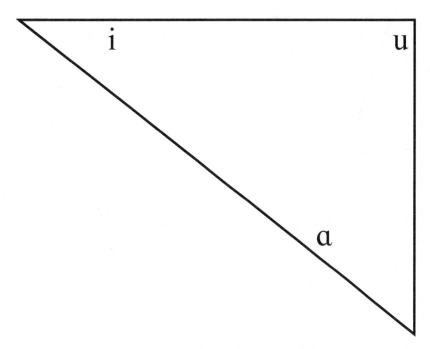

**Figure 7–2.** Vowel triangle with English /ɑ/.

When clients practice producing these sounds, they can see the typical boundaries of the world's languages, giving them some fixed reference points when adding the other vowels. At this point, SLPs can explain that the chart is designed to show tongue position, with the left representing the front of the mouth. The /i/ vowel would therefore be produced with the tongue in a high, front position, while /a/ would be low. Although most people have a difficult time feeling where their tongue is in their mouth, these gross indicators are useful for building awareness. The vowels are nearly universal and are also highly distinguishable, so clients should be able to feel the major differences in tongue position that creates these vastly different shapes.

We can also adjust the triangle slightly, as shown in Figure 7–2, to show the relative positions of the English vowels because the English /ɑ/ vowel is probably different than the more common /a/ found in other languages. Keep in mind that the range of differences at the bottom is smaller than at the top, which explains why a quadrilateral and not a square is used when including all of the vowels.

To develop an understanding of how these vowels work, clients can also be asked why doctors have patients say "ah" and not "ee" during an examination, and they should immediately grasp that /ɑ/ has the widest mouth opening in English. Clients can also experiment with moving the tongue further out from each of these vowels to start to feel the point at which it no longer becomes possible to produce a sound. Next, we can add the /æ/ vowel to create the frontiers of the English system, and this is shown in Figure 7–3.

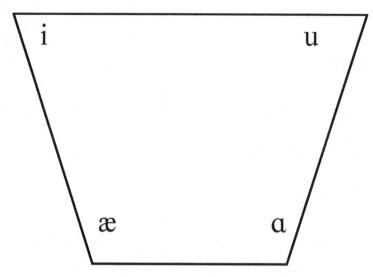

**Figure 7–3.** Corner vowels of the English quadrilateral.

The /æ/ vowel sound is rarer in the world's languages compared to /a,i,u/, and it is a common target in accent modification. Clinicians should highlight awareness of this phoneme early because it helps establish how the vowel boundaries of our inventory may differ from the client's language. Much of the work that clinicians do with this vowel sound involves having the client use a lowered jaw, so depict a visual representation of this phoneme at the bottom of the quadrilateral.

The final vowel is in the mid-central range, where we find the /ʌ,ə/, as shown in Figure 7–4. One way to introduce this vowel is to model it and have clients try to identify

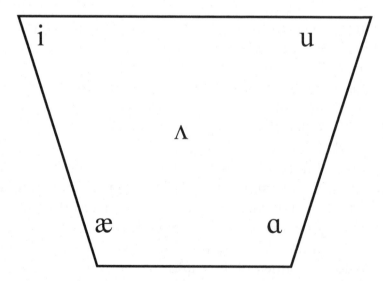

**Figure 7–4.** English vowel frontiers with /ʌ/.

where in the chart it might belong, as this type of elicitation technique will improve clients' internalization of the information. It can also simply be presented to the client, and in either case, it helps to point out that this space is not as commonly used around the world.

SLPs tend to have mixed thoughts regarding the use of the /ʌ,ə/ symbols, so let's review the reasons why English has two symbols for vowels that have very similar characteristics. By convention, the /ʌ/ (called the turned v or wedge, among other things) is used to transcribe a stressed vowel, and its counterpart, /ə/ (the schwa), is used for unstressed syllables. When I teach undergraduate phonetics, the most frequently asked question is why we have two symbols, since students complain that they cannot hear the difference between the two vowel sounds. I have found that the easiest way to explain it is to tell students not to try to hear a difference between the vowels, but to view the schwa as a phonological symbol designed to show how vowels are reduced in English. While it is certainly important to convey the concept of the schwa and its role in reductions to non-native clients, they do not need to learn the conventions of English transcription, so many SLPs simply merge the two symbols to avoid distraction. The decision about whether to use the /ʌ,ə/ or just the /ə/ comes down to personal preference, taking into account a client's overall level of proficiency, general grasp of linguistic concepts, the amount of time available for training, and any other pertinent factors.

Once the parameters of the English vowel system are established, SLPs can review key vowels, keeping in mind that clients may need time to establish connections between the sounds, symbols, and physical movements needed to produce them. Additional vowels can now be added to the chart. Clinicians can use principles of contrastive analysis to determine which vowels are most useful to highlight. Figure 7–5 illustrates the monophthongs of American English.

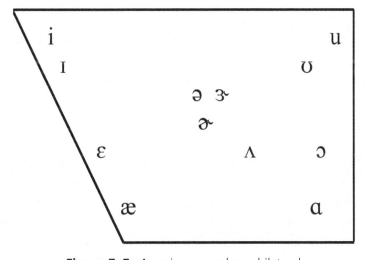

**Figure 7–5.** American vowel quadrilateral.

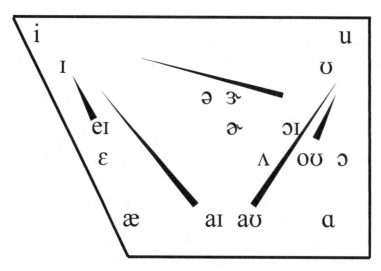

**Figure 7–6.** American vowel quadrilateral with diphthongs.

**Table 7–1.** American Vowels in Words

| beat /bit/ | | boot /but/ |
|---|---|---|
| bit /bɪt/ | | book /bʊk/ |
| bait /beɪt/ | Burt /bɝt/ | boat /boʊt/ |
| bet /bɛt/ | but /bʌt/ | caught /kɑt/ or /kɔt/ |
| bat /bæt/ | | cot /kɑt/ |

Adding the diphthongs of American English requires showing some movement through the vowel space, as shown in Figure 7–6. Another useful way of categorizing the vowels is to use model words, such as those shown in Table 7–1. Note that many speakers of American English from areas including the west coast and Midwest have merged the vowels of caught and cot and pronounce both with a vowel close to the /ɑ/.

Table 7–1 may be more client-friendly than a traditional vowel quadrilateral, and the advantage of using model words is that clients may be able to memorize the vowel and its position. In this type of chart, the context /bVt/ is used wherever possible for consistency, with the exception of *caught* and *cot*, which are the most widely cited examples to illustrate the vowel sound merger. For clinicians working with clients on a dialect of American English that lacks the /ɔ/, the word *bought* can be substituted to preserve the /bVt/ context. Another useful set of keywords comes from J. C. Wells in his book *Accents of English* (1982). Wells used a system he called "lexical sets," which have proven to be an excellent way to analyzing dialects. Table 7–2 shows the keywords from Wells' lexical sets organized by tongue position.

**Table 7–2.** Lexical Set Keywords

| fleece /flis/ | | goose /gus/ |
|---|---|---|
| kit /kɪt/ | | foot /fʊt/ |
| face /feɪs/ | nurse /nɝs/ | goat /goʊt/ |
| dress /drɛs/ | strut /strʌt/ | North /nɔɚθ/ |
| bath /bæθ/ | | palm /pɑm/ |

**Table 7–3.** Vowel Length Contexts

| Context | Example | Vowel Length |
|---|---|---|
| Preceding an unvoiced consonant | beat | shortest |
| Preceding a voiced consonant | bead | longer |
| Open syllable | bee | longest |

## Vowel Length

In some languages, such as Hungarian, vowel length is phonemic, so the words *örült* (he was glad), pronounced as /ørylt/ and *örült* (crazy) pronounced as /øːrylt/ differ only in terms of the length of the first vowel. In English, vowel length is allophonic and depends on four main factors (Ladefoged & Disner, 2012):

1. The vowel itself (e.g., /i/ is longer than /ɪ/)
2. Stress, with stressed vowels longer than unstressed vowels
3. Number of syllables, with vowels in shorter words held longer than those in longer words
4. Phonetic context

Of these factors, the most important for non-native speakers is context, so clinicians should develop awareness of how vowel length relates to word shape. Table 7–3 shows the relative lengths of the /i/ vowel in monosyllabic words.

It is important to introduce this concept to clients when working with both vowels and consonants since it plays a key role in distinguishing between final voiced and unvoiced stops and also influences the length of final fricatives. Often, when working with consonants, it is important to distinguish the vowel length difference and focus clients' attention on it. When working with vowels, however, clinicians often contrast two vowels in minimal pairs of words that feature them in the same phonetic context, so it is important to prevent clients from attempting to use length as the key differentiator. For example, clients may work on the vowels /ɪ/ and /i/ with the minimal pair *bit/beat*. Even though the /i/ is generally longer than the /ɪ/, if a client stretches out the /i/ in the word *beat* it will not sound natural because the phonetic context mandates shortening of both vowels. Clinicians should therefore be on the lookout for contexts which will allow them to exaggerate distinctions, but they need to use caution when emphasizing it to produce a contrast between vowels if the context would not normally produce a longer vowel.

### Tense and Lax Vowels

The tense/lax distinction in English differs from that of many other languages, and this can be problematic for non-native speakers. The terms *tense* and *lax* distinguish pairs of vowels in English that are made with similar degrees of height, backness, and rounding, but differ articulatorily in terms of muscle tension and length. Some of the differences are phonological, and some phoneticians refer to them as free and checked vowels because of the types of syllables in which they can occur. Free (tense) vowels can occur in CV words (or any other stressed open syllables), while lax (checked) vowels cannot. This information may be useful in developing general awareness. Clients can be given vowels and asked to come up with a CV word containing the vowel to focus attention on this distinction, but in the end, clients probably need to spend most of their time and energy working simply on how to produce the lax vowels themselves.

Lax vowels are especially troublesome because there are many minimal pairs featuring everyday words where the distinction can easily create opportunities for misunderstandings. If a non-native speaker pronounces /ɪ/ as /i/ then "I live here" may come out as "I leave here." Although American English contains five lax vowels (ɪ,ɛ,æ,ʌ,ʊ), only three of them have tense counterparts that create difficult vowel pairs for non-native speakers. (/i,ɪ/, /eɪ,ɛ/, and /u,ʊ/). These contrasts involve vowels that are made in a similar space, so clients have to discern a difference that may be imperceptible to them at first. Pointing out that the lax vowel sounds are made in a slightly lower and more centralized place may be of little help when working with non-native speakers, so clinicians tend to focus on the difference in the feeling of muscle tension and on vowel length. When focusing on vowel pairs such as /i,ɪ/ in isolation, clinicians can highlight which muscle groups in the face and neck are involved and show the increased spreading of the lips for /i/, but the pairs cannot be contrasted in open syllables because the lax vowels sounds do not occur in those contexts. To take advantage of the potential increased lengthening for the tense vowels, use minimal pairs that end in voiced consonants, so *bead/bid* is a better place to start than *beat/bit*.

### The Schwa and Reduced Vowels

One of the most important differences between the English vowel system and that of many other languages is the tendency to reduce unstressed vowels. Reduced vowels sound weaker and are more centralized. If we compare the vowel sounds in the related words *finite* and *infinite*, we can see this effect. The word *finite* is stressed on the first syllable and has two clear vowels /faɪnaɪt/, but when we add the prefix to form the antonym, the stress shifts to the first syllable, and the two following vowels sounds become reduced to

/ˈɪnfənət/. If you feel that you are producing one or both of the last two vowels as /ɪ/ or another more central allophone, you are probably right. While the schwa is the most common reduced vowel sound in English, /ɪ/ is almost always a possible substitution in unstressed syllables. The shift from a full vowel sound (in this case the diphthong /aɪ/) to the schwa is a hallmark feature of English. In comparison, the Spanish cognate *infinito* /infinito/ features the same /i/ vowel phoneme three times because no matter what happens to the stress in a Spanish word, the vowel will retain its qualities. Clients who do not reduce their vowels are likely to sound excessively clear, as if they are over-pronouncing everything, and they will not sound natural.

Due to the prevalence of this feature of English, the schwa is the most common vowel sound in our language, and it is worth a significant investment of time unless clients naturally reduce vowels. Since the middle and central vowel space is less commonly used in vowel inventories of the world, clients may need some training in how to produce the schwa. Clinicians can demonstrate the /ʌ/ and have clients work at producing a relaxed neutral vowel sound. The schwa itself is phonological, so it cannot truly be produced in isolation since it only occurs when it is not stressed. In a sense, it is like the principle in quantum mechanics that observing something changes it, so there is really no way for a speaker to isolate a schwa. The point of the schwa is that the spotlight is always off it, even though some might consider it the star of our vowel system.

Key to assisting clients in generalizing reduced vowels is developing their awareness of them, and one way to do this is to simply have them identify schwas in common words or names. Often, the name of the country they come from is pronounced with a schwa, so you might start with a comparison of the way a client says the name of their country in their language versus English. A Brazilian client might produce their country's name in Portuguese as /bɾaziʊ/, which can be contrasted with English /bɹəzɪl/, where the first vowel is reduced. Walking clients through several words that exemplify reduction brings its prevalence to their attention. In some cases, variations in the English pronunciation of a client's name, compared to their native language, can also highlight this effect, as in /məɹiə/ versus /maria/ for *Maria*. In languages that share a large number of cognates with English (such as the Romance languages), it can be especially important to heighten awareness of important differences in how words are produced in each language. The following is a sample exercise designed to guide clients in identifying schwas:

Circle the schwas in the following words and names, as they are pronounced in English:

| California | Maria | Florida | organization |
| hippopotamus | banana | Isabella | assistant |
| economical | delicious | animal | democracy |

Because schwas and reductions are such important features of English, it must be highlighted when working with vowels, but often the best practice opportunities come up when working on suprasegmentals, such as stress and connected speech. For example, clients need to understand that the difference between word pairs such as object (n.) and object (v.) relates not only to the shift in stress from the first to the second syllable, but also to the reduction that occurs in the first vowel. When clients work on connected speech, they typically need to reduce the vowels in function words, so it is important to have some experience with the schwa when they work on producing /əv/, or even /ə/. The schwa also opens the door to working on vowel syncope, in which the vowel disappears altogether.

## Gliding

English vowels may also differ from their counterparts in other languages by their gliding. To highlight this distinction, compare a word such as *see* /si/ in English to the Spanish word *sí* /si/ since they are transcribed broadly in the same manner. When we produce these words, we can hear that the English vowel is longer and has some gliding. If we listen to a native speaker say this word in isolation, there is an echo effect that almost makes it sound as if the /i/ is repeated. Although by convention we don't transcribe words with /j/ word finally in English, we can think of this as more of an /iʲ/ sound, compared to the clipped pure /i/ sound in the Spanish word. In much the same way, when we produce words that end in a rounded vowel, we hear a slight /w/ glide. When we compare the Spanish word *tú* (/tu/) with the English word *too* (/tu/) we hear much more gliding and rounding in the English version. Table 7–4 can help clients identify these differences.

## Roundedness and Lip Position

The rounding effect mentioned in the word *too* highlights another allophonic difference that is key to natural vowel productions. In some languages, roundness is contrastive, so the French minimal pairs *si* (/si/; if) and *su* (/sy/; known) both feature high front vowels made in the same place, but the roundness of /y/ distinguishes these words. German has similar pairs such as *für* [fyːɐ̯] (for) and *vier* [fiːɐ̯] (four). In English, roundness is not phonemic, but we do round several of our monophthongs and diphthongs, and the presence or extent of rounding is important. If we compare an English speaker saying the word *no* /noʊ/ with the diphthong with the Spanish word *no* /no/ with its monophthong, besides the movement of the vowel, a key difference is the roundness at the end of the word. Rounding is not phonemic in English, so clinicians may be less familiar with it. Clients may produce vowels that differ in roundness from their English counterparts, and the SLP can help identify the problem and train clients to avoid it.

Lip position, while not phonemic in English, can nonetheless help clients sound more natural and produce vowels that are more typical of native speakers' models. Generally,

**Table 7–4.** Vowel Gliding

| English | Spanish/Italian/Other language? |
|---|---|
| see = [siʲ] | si  = [si] |
| two = [tuʷ] | tu = [tu] |

the most important distinctions to highlight are the spread lips in words such as *me* or *my*, the rounded lips in words such as *do* and *go*, and the pursed lips in words such as *book* or *were*. When working individually with clients, ask them to use a mirror while producing model words and to describe the shape of their mouth. In pair and group work, clients can work together to identify these forms. In developing awareness of the spread lip pattern, I often ask clients why English speakers say "cheese" when taking photographs, and hopefully they answer that it is to guarantee a good smile, as opposed to saying a word like *dog*, that would produce strange-looking pictures. Ask clients to share the word from their language that is used when taking pictures; it usually contains the /i/ vowel. Koreans, for example, say "kimchi" [kim.tɕʰi]. When clients identify rounding in words with back vowels, point out how this might differ from their language, especially if it is an Indo-European language that features English cognates. It can help to imitate a less rounded version of these vowels to heighten awareness. Finally, when working with the pursed lip shape of vowels, such as /ʊ,ɝ/, ask clients to describe the shape and they may come up with answers such as a duck's beak, or a trumpet. Awareness of lip position is also important when working on secondary articulations involved in consonants such as /ʃ/.

The neutral lip position in words with the mid-central vowel phonemes, and the wide open lips of words with low back vowel sounds are best addressed in terms of jaw position, as opposed to labiality. Understanding of jaw movement is handy to distinguish some difficult pairs such as /ɛ,æ/, and to make sure that clients are in a neutral position for /ə,ʌ/. Some clients have a reduced range of jaw movement, whether from speaking their native language or their own style of speaking. Clinicians can help clients enunciate more clearly by using a mirror, or even having them place their fingers or a sterilized item such as a thick plastic rod in their mouth to focus on extending their jaw.

### Diphthongs

Most phoneticians consider American English to have five diphthongs, as outlined in Figure 7–6. Some phoneticians use a three-diphthong system to analyze English (Yavas, 2016), and they remove /oʊ/ and /eɪ/ because there is less of a change in the overall vowel, and they can be represented with the symbols /o,e/. In accent modification, the five-diphthong system is more commonly used because it heightens clients' awareness of the gliding effects that occur in these vowels. For example, /oʊ/ and /o/ can be contrasted for a Spanish-speaking client to highlight the difference between a native Spanish model of a word such as *taco* as /tako/ versus a typical English-speaker's pronunciation of this loanword as /takoʊ/.

### Rhoticity, Nasality, Voicing

A prominent feature of American vowels is their rhoticity, which makes them stand out in comparison to those of most versions of English spoken in other countries and many dialects of American English (such as Boston, New York, or Southern English) spoken throughout the United States. Rhoticity refers to r-coloring and the r-controlled vowels of

American English are also rare in most other languages of the world. While the citation form of the word *teacher* in American English is pronounced /tiʧɚ/, many speakers of other English dialects and many non-native speakers acquiring English produce it as /tiʧə/, or in some cases, with a distorted postvocalic /ɹ/. In contrast to other distinctions, such as tenseness/laxness, height, or backness, a lack of rhoticity should not lead to significantly reduced intelligibility since it is so common among the dialects of English and such a common error pattern for non-native speakers. On the other hand, a lack of rhoticity may set non-natives apart when they communicate in American English, and acquiring r-colored vowels helps them sound more natural in most parts of the United States. For this reason, clinicians work on producing natural r-colored vowels with many of their clients. Much of the previous discussion on producing the consonantal /ɹ/ of English applies here, and in general, clinicians will rely on feedback and modeling to help clients acquire these vowels. The schwar /ɚ/ is the rhotic counterpart to the schwa and phonologically, it represents vowel reduction in unstressed syllables. If clients are able to produce a good approximation of the /ɝ/, it is rarely a problem for them to create the unstressed version.

Nasality is not phonemic in English, but it is an allophonic feature of English vowels that can influence perception of clients' naturalness. An allophonic rule of English is that vowels are nasalized when they proceed a nasal in the same syllable, so the word *fin* in English can be transcribed narrowly as [fɪ̃n], while the word *fit* would be [fɪt]. The amount of nasality varies among dialects of English, and clinicians must use their judgment to guide clients toward producing an appropriate level. In some languages, such as French, Portuguese, and possibly Polish, nasality is phonemic. For example, Portuguese has the minimal pairs *lá* (/lɐ/; here) and *lã* (/lɐ̃/; wool), where the only difference is the nasality of the vowel. Clients whose native language has prominent nasal vowels often produce English vowels with excessive nasality, so it is typical for Brazilian clients to produce the word *but* as [bɐ̃t] even though the native English version features a purely oral vowel.

Although all of the vowels of English are voiced phonemically, there are some situations in which allophonic unvoiced vowels emerge. For example, in the word *potato*, the schwa vowel in the first syllable might become devoiced because it is unstressed and between unvoiced stops. Some languages, such as Japanese, also have unvoiced vowels as allophonic variations. Clinicians should be aware of possible allophonic mismatches when working with clients who speak these languages.

### Coarticulation

To demonstrate the effects of coarticulation, have clients prepare to say a word featuring a back vowel (without saying it), such as *goose*, and then prepare to say a minimal pair containing a front vowel, such as *geese* (again, without actually saying it). Point to the written form of the word or pictures to prompt clients to say one and then the other. By doing this exercise in silence, clients can see that lip position changes drastically even though the sounds begin with the same consonant /g/ and not a vowel. The purpose is to develop awareness that words and phrases are not produced by stringing together disconnected phonemes. Speech consists of connected sounds, and when sounds come together, there are coarticulation effects which produce allophones. Clients will learn that they may hear slight differences in the way a particular vowel is realized in a context, but that this represents an allophonic difference, and this will help them develop categorical perception of the phonemes. It is typical for clients to have difficulty believing that two words are actually produced with the same vowel phoneme because of these effects; they may not hear that words such as *pit* and *pill* are produced with the same /ɪ/ phoneme because of the retraction effect of the /l/ in *pill*, for example. In some cases, a neutralized context may cause the vowel to land somewhere in between two phonemes, and clients should be aware of this effect as well. The vowels in *keen* and *kin* should be easier to identify compared to the vowel in *king* which features a neutralized context. While *keen* and *kin* are minimal pairs, producing *king* as /kiŋ/ or /kɪŋ/ would not produce words with different meanings, and it is likely that the actual vowel sound falls somewhere in between the two pronunciations.

## American English and Other Dialects

When working with vowels, bear in mind that dialects of English are generally distinguished by their vowel systems, as opposed to consonantal variations, and this has several key implications. First, clients' accents may be influenced by other versions of English depending on where they have lived or which version of English was taught in their country. A client producing the word *not* as [nɒt] uses a vowel sound found in British Received Pronunciation, but not in American English, and even in the United States, the word might be pronounced as [nɔt], [nat], [nɑt] or something in between. Clinicians should be on the lookout for influences of other English dialects and then work with the client to determine which vowel system should be the target. Clients can also be informed of these dialectal differences to help them code switch as desired. In some cases clients are also influenced by dialects of American English that feature different vowels than the clinician uses.

Perhaps the most typical vowel mismatch is the use of the /ɔ/ vowel sound since it tends to be merged with the /ɑ/ vowel sound in many versions of American English. At SDSU, many undergraduates are initially confused when they see this symbol in their textbooks because of its relative scarcity in California English. Clinicians should develop a good awareness of how to use this vowel in American English, and then determine how to best approach it with clients. A client living in California, for example, may wish to speak a version of English without this phoneme, while a client in New York might choose to adopt it. Clinicians should also feel comfortable with their own dialect and can focus exclusively on that when training, but it might be beneficial to point out key differences in dialects of American English clients are likely to encounter. Clinicians should not feel that they must speak a particular dialect to be successful, and if a clinician produces vowel sounds in a slightly different way from the way some other native speakers do (e.g., lack of a distinction between /ɪ,ɛ/ before nasals, which is common in the South, or the use of two different vowel sounds in the words *marry* and *merry*, which is common on the East Coast), they can point these differences out to clients who aim to acquire the typical vowel phonemes of American English. On a final note, clients should be made aware that books and materials from other English-speaking countries will most likely feature significant vowel differences, especially in terms of rhoticity, for example, they may find a pronunciation guide listing the pronunciation of "bird" as /bɜːd/, and this may be misleading if they are aiming for a more American sounding accent.

## Typical Targets

Typical of Germanic languages, English has a higher than average number of vowel phonemes in its inventory, so it is likely that clients will need to acquire a handful of new vowels in order to communicate effectively. Nevertheless, as outlined in the section on target selection, clinicians should weigh many considerations when developing training priorities. While the /ʊ/ phoneme is relatively uncommon and often presents challenges for non-native speakers, there are only a limited number of minimal pairs contrasting this vowel with its tense counterpart, /u/, and these phonemes are unlikely to lead to serious miscommunications. The vowel sound itself is also not found in many English words, although those that use it are high frequency (e.g., could, would, should, good). If a client produces the sentence, "I could call you later," as "I cooed call you later," it is improbable that the message would be lost. On the other hand, if a client produces, "I live here," as "I leave here," there is a good chance of a misunderstanding.

### /i/ vs. /ɪ/

Due to a spacing principle, the tense/lax distinction is unlikely to occur in many of the languages of our clients which have five or fewer vowels. In addition, because the tense/lax /i,ɪ/ pair tends to be problematic for many Romance language speakers, and since the United States has many immigrants from Spanish-speaking countries, even lay people identify this as a typical error pattern for many non-native speakers from those countries. This pair is considered to have a high functional load, and the number of minimal pairs featuring those two vowel sounds is said to number above 300 (Shakhbagova & University of Southern California, 2008). In addition, while the /i/ is a common vowel in English, coming in fourth place, its more difficult lax counterpart ranks even higher at second place (Edwards, 1992).

As the /i/ vowel is extremely common in the world's languages, there is generally no need to practice this phoneme, and instead, clinicians will most likely target its lax counterpart. Nevertheless, clients often begin overgeneralizing the /ɪ/ on their path to mastering it, which can lead to misunderstandings and even embarrassment, since the minimal pairs featuring the lax counterparts for the tense vowels in the words *sheet*, *beach*, and *peace* are mildly taboo words. *Sheet* and *beach* in particular are frequently cited by non-native speakers as troublesome words due to anxiety about producing the wrong vowel.

Contrasting it with the client's presumably accurate /i/ is often the first step to producing an accurate /ɪ/. The /i/ vowel should already be in the client's phonemic inventory, and generally the only area of concern is the gliding factor that differentiates it from the client's native version. Clients should be made aware of the glide effect and practice saying CV words ending in /i/ to make sure they produce it accurately. As a prompt, they can listen for a word, and then repeat the word with a noticeable repetition of the /i/. For example, to produce a natural English version of the word *see*, clients can produce something akin to [siʲiː] and then fade the repeated vowel until it becomes just a glide. Even if clients cannot produce a completely natural English /i/, their native /i/ provides a good reference point for examining the contrast with its lax counterpart. Cue clients to produce the /i/ and feel the tension at the root of their tongue by putting their hands around their chin, lips, and upper neck. When the client produces the /ɪ/, they should strive to feel some of the muscles going limp, and they should attempt to produce a more neutral vowel sound. Although the tongue is lowered and centralized slightly, it is unlikely that clients will be helped by a conceptual understanding of this, so feeling the pressure is more productive. Clinicians should model the lip position since the /i/ is produced with spread lips while the /ɪ/ has the lips in a more neutral, partially-spread position. Clients should monitor their production with a mirror to see this. Finally, the extra length and the echo effect of the slight /j/ glide in /i/ can help clients distinguish a difference. Clinicians can start with minimal pairs such as *bead*/*bid* or *scene*/*sin* that produce longer versions of the vowels and highlight the contrast, but it is important to keep clients from relying on the length distinction too much or they will produce words such as *seat* or *feet* with excessively lengthened vowels, when the final unvoiced consonant requires a shorter vowel. Appendix 7–4 contains minimal pairs in words and sentences for use with clients.

### /eɪ/ vs. /ɛ/

This is the second common tense/lax pair that often causes problems. In this case, clients typically have /e/ in their inventory and /ɛ/ is less common. The client's /e/, however, will most likely be a monophthong, so it is important to call attention to the movement that occurs to produce the English /eɪ/, especially in stressed syllables. Clinicians can provide models of this sound, exaggerating the transition and perhaps drawing it out and pausing along the way to show the path of the vowel sound. Clinicians can learn to produce a monopthongized version of the diphthong in stressed syllables to imitate a client's native language, and then see if clients can catch this purposely less natural production when the clinician reads words aloud. The lengthening, gliding, and lip spreading that occurs with /eɪ/ can be highlighted as they were above for the /i/.

Once again, even if the client does not produce an entirely accurate /eɪ/, the /e/ from the client's language (especially since it is essentially an allophonic variation of the diphthong in English) should still serve as a good reference point to establish the lax counterpart /ɛ/. Clinicians can use some of the same cues as discussed for /i/ versus /ɪ/ since /ɛ/ is also produced in a slightly lower, more central area than its counterpart. Clinician should also emphasize proprioception of the lessened muscle tension for the /ɛ/.

### /ʊ/ vs. /u/

This represents our final tense/lax pair, and it is clearly the least important due to its low functional load. Clinicians may in fact struggle to come up with minimal pairs using words that clients are familiar with. Some of the more common minimal pairs used to contrast these vowels are *hood/who'd, could/cooed, should/shoed.* The chances for misunderstandings are greatly diminished for these pairs in comparison to /i,ɪ/ minimal pairs. As with /i,e/, a phoneme close to the tense /u/ vowel is common in the world's languages, so it will generally not be difficult for clients to produce. In some cases, a client's rounding may be different from English rounding, as with certain speakers of Japanese where the /u/ in its five-vowel inventory is produced more like an [ɯ], (i.e., with less rounding). The /u/ therefore serves as a good anchor for production of the /ʊ/, which in keeping with the previous pattern for tense versus lax vowels, is placed lower and more centrally. The rounding of the /u/ can be contrasted with the pursing of the lips for /ʊ/, and perhaps most importantly, clients can focus on producing the /ʊ/ with less muscular tension. Although work on distinguishing the /ʊ/ from the /u/ is clearly less urgent than the need to create clear contrasts between /i,ɪ/ and /eɪ,ɛ/, a case can be made for working on accurately producing this phoneme because it occurs in high-frequency words, such as the modals *should, would, could,* and *look,* as well as the frequently used *good,* all of which are in the 200 most common words of English (Kress, 2014).

## /ɔ/ vs. /ɑ/

This is another example of a potential vowel pair that may be of little value in training. Although clinicians may choose to teach the English /ɔ/ and /ɑ/ vowel sounds as separate phonemes depending on the target dialect of American English, these vowel sounds appear to be in the process of merging in the United States, and in many parts of the country (including California) the /ɔ/ vowel sound is rare. Potential minimal pairs could be *caught/cot, stock/stalk,* or *collar/caller,* but clinicians whose dialect does not distinguish between these words and who are working in regions of the country where the /ɔ/ is not phonemic are advised to avoid introducing this distinction to clients unless they specifically request it.

## /ɑ/ vs. /æ/

Difficulties with this contrast result mainly from substitution of the /ɑ/ for the /æ/ since a client's L1 phonemic inventory is more likely to contain the former than the latter. While most languages have a vowel similar to the /ɑ/, it is likely to be more forward and may be represented as an /a/. Due to the reduced space at the bottom of the vowel quadrilateral, this distinction should be less consequential, so a client's intelligibility will probably not be greatly impacted by producing /ɑ/ as /a/. The /æ/ vowel, on the other hand, is relatively rare in other languages, so clients may back this vowel until it lands in a zone they are comfortable with. This contrast has a relatively high functional load, as evidenced by minimal pairs such as *backs/box, add/odd,* and *stack/stock.* The /æ/ is the third most common vowel phoneme of English and the /ɑ/ comes in fifth (Edwards, 1992), so both vowels have relatively high frequencies. Since both vowel sounds are produced low in the mouth, clinicians can guide clients to move the tongue forward without changing the position of the jaw.

## /ɛ/ vs. /æ/

The challenges arising from this pair result primarily from the rarity of both phonemes in the languages of the world. Typical five-vowel inventories contain /a,i,e,o,u/, so many clients need to acquire both of these vowels without a vowel from their native language to use as an anchor. On a positive note, these two phonemes have the advantage of differing primarily in terms of height, so clinicians can easily demonstrate the main difference between them by placing a hand under the jaw and producing minimal pairs featuring these words. Figure 7–7 shows a client following her clinician's visual prompt to have her jaw in the right position for the /ɛ/ vowel. The clinician can then focus awareness on how the jaw drops down. Figure 7–8 shows the client following her clinician's prompt to produce the /æ/ with the jaw in a lower position.

Although the order is not important, clinicians can start with a word such as *bend*, which contains the /ɛ/ vowel, and then produce the word *band*, which features the /æ/ vowel. By placing a hand under the jaw, the clinician can draw attention to the lower position of the tongue as the jaw drops to produce the second vowel. Clients can then use a mirror and imitate these productions while concentrating on the visual feedback of their reflection. The advantage of working with these two front vowels, which are similar in most ways apart from height, should be apparent since they can be demonstrated well

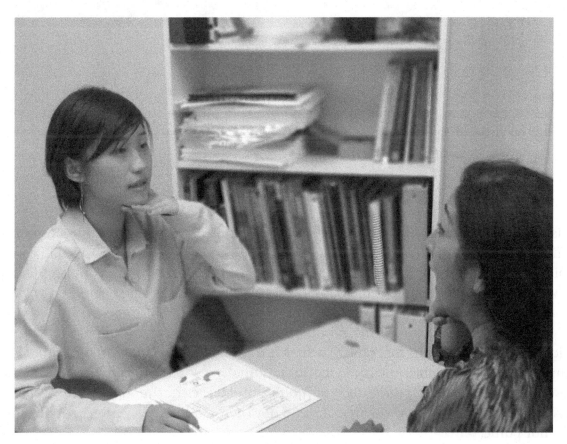

**Figure 7–7.** Modeling /ɛ/.

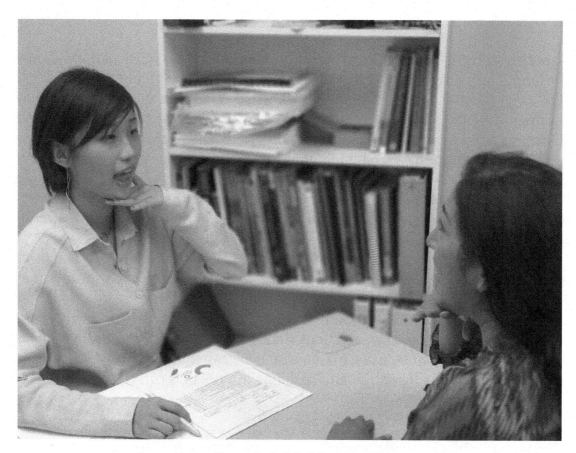

**Figure 7–8.** Modeling /æ/.

visually. Clients tend to develop awareness of how to produce the lower vowel relatively quickly because of the visual feedback. Appendix 7–5 contains minimal pairs in words and sentences designed to target these two vowels.

## /ɑ/ vs. /ʌ/

This troublesome pair differs in terms of both height and backness and is especially difficult for clients because fewer languages feature vowel sounds in the mid-central region. While frequency of the /ʌ/ comes in at 12th place among the vowels of English (Edwards, 1992), its phonological counterpart (the schwa) is the most common vowel of all, and the /ɑ/, which non-natives often substitute for it, is the fifth most common vowel (Edwards, 1992). Estimates of the number of minimal pairs are in the 170 plus range (Higgins, J., Minimal pairs for English), which is a strong indicator of high functional load. Clinicians should be able to easily identify minimal pairs featuring relatively common words, such as *come/calm*, *stuck/stock*, or *rub/rob*, and it is clear that a non-native speaker saying, "There's a bomb over there," instead of "There's a bum over there," might cause a minor panic.

Clinicians can shape clients' /ɑ/ from its equivalent in the client's language, but it is generally more important to focus on production of a clear contrast with the /ʌ/. While the /ɑ/ vowel can serve as a reference to produce an accurate /ʌ/, this will often be an arduous process since many vowel inventories are vacant in the mid-central region, and clients may have difficulty perceiving vowels in this space or producing them accurately. Production of the /ʌ/, while essential on its own, is also the key to its unstressed counterpart, the schwa, which is extremely important in creating the natural, reduced vowels of English. Clinicians generally point out to clients that this vowel is produced in a neutral position, with the tongue right in the middle of the mouth and the lips parted slightly and relaxed. It may help to work on this sound in isolation and see if clients can come close through modeling and feedback. Clinicians can point out to clients that this is the "thinking sound" that native speakers use when they are trying to buy time or unable to answer a question. When asked to name the capital of Zimbabwe, a speaker of English might answer with a lengthy /ʌː/ while racking their brains. Pointing this out to clients creates an opportunity to develop awareness when they hear native speakers produce these filler vowels throughout the day.

Directing clients to move the tongue in various directions may not be effective in and of itself due to poor proprioception, but clinicians can shape clients' productions by indicating when the vowel is approaching the correct space. Minimal pairs are also effective for highlighting this distinction, and they can be used to raise awareness and perception through auditory discrimination and improve accuracy and naturalness in clients' productions. Clients often tend to substitute the lower /a/ or /ɑ/ vowels, but in some cases, clients favor an /o/ or /ɔ/ due to spelling interference. A speaker might therefore typically produce *brother* as /bɹaðɚ/, but if a client produces it as /bɹoðɚ/, it is most likely because the word is spelled with an *o*. In that case, it is important to work on improving awareness, monitoring vowel sounds carefully, and relying less on orthography.

When working with some of vowel sounds that tend to be more difficult for non-native-speaking clients, it helps to work with minimal sets once a level of confidence has been attained. Table 7–5 is an example of a minimal set that would target the /ʌ/ and its typical substitutions.

**Table 7–5.** /oʊ, ʌ, ɑ/ Minimal Sets

|   | **A. /oʊ/** | **B. /ʌ/** | **C. /ɑ/** |
|---|---|---|---|
| 1 | robe | rub | rob |
| 2 | comb | come | calm |
| 3 | pope | pup | pop |
| 4 | wrote | rut | rot |
| 5 | goat | gut | got |

We can also branch out to add the /æ/ vowel sound as shown in Table 7–6, and this will help clients focus on two problematic sounds, /æ, ʌ/, along with a typical substitution for them, /ɑ/. Sentence minimal pairs featuring these vowels are shown in Table 7–7. Or we can challenge clients with a set of four or more vowel sounds to test their skills, as shown in Table 7–8. Appendix 7–6 provides additional sets of these vowels for use with clients.

**Table 7–6.** /æ, ʌ, ɑ/ Minimal Sets

|   | A. /æ/ | B. /ʌ/ | C. /ɑ/ |
|---|--------|--------|--------|
| 1 | cab    | cub    | cob    |
| 2 | bag    | bug    | bog    |
| 3 | sack   | suck   | sock   |
| 4 | stack  | stuck  | stock  |
| 5 | cap    | cup    | cop    |

**Table 7–7.** /æ, ʌ, ɑ/ Minimal Set Sentences

|   | A. /æ/ | B. /ʌ/ | C. /ɑ/ |
|---|--------|--------|--------|
| 1 | The caps are there. | The cups are there. | The cops are there. |
| 2 | The cat is on the rug. | The cut is on the rug. | The cot is on the rug. |
| 3 | Did you see the bag? | Did you see the bug? | Did you see the bog? |
| 4 | Is that Dan? | Is that done? | Is that Don? |
| 5 | Where is the mask? | Where is the musk? | Where is the mosque? |

**Table 7–8.** /ɛ, æ, ʌ, ɑ/ Minimal Sets

|   | A. /ɛ/ | B. /æ/ | C. /ʌ/ | D. /ɑ/ |
|---|--------|--------|--------|--------|
| 1 | den    | Dan    | done   | Don    |
| 2 | net    | gnat   | nut    | knot   |
| 3 | flex   | flax   | flux   | flocks |
| 4 | tech   | tack   | tuck   | talk   |
| 5 | pen    | pan    | pun    | pawn   |

# References

Edwards, H. T. (1992). *Applied phonetics: Instructor's manual*. San Diego, CA: Singular Publishing Group.

Higgins, J. Minimal pairs for English RP [Web Resource]. Retrieved from: https://minimal -pairs.000webhostapp.com/minimal.html

Kress, J. E. (2014). *The ESL/ELL teacher's book of lists*. New York, NY: John Wiley & Sons.

Ladefoged, P. (2005). *Vowels and consonants: An introduction to the sounds of languages*. Malden, MA: Blackwell Publishing

Ladefoged, P., & Johnson, K. (2015). *A course in phonetics*.

Ladefoged, P., & Disner, S. F. (2012). *Vowels and consonants*. Malden, MA: Wiley-Blackwell.

Shakhbagova, J., & University of Southern California (2008). *Correcting errors in pronunciation: A resource manual for ESL, EFL teachers*. Los Angeles, CA: Figueroa Press.

Wells, J. C. (1982). *Accents of English. Volume 1: An Introduction*. Cambridge, UK: Cambridge University Press

Yavas, M. (2016). *Applied English phonology*. Hoboken, NJ: John Wiley & Sons Inc.

# 7-1

# Vowel Contrast Sentences Worksheet

1. While Tim was on the team he was seeking a sick sheep to put on the ship.
2. I met my mate and he led me to the red gate, where we laid a wet mat.
3. Bess and Beth wasted time at the west gate. They played chess and ate cheese.
4. The cat and man get gas with dad. They beg for bags and bend the bands.
5. Ed said he was sad and added he was mad. I was glad he had said that then.
6. I patted the pet in the pot with Don and Dan in the den. "That was odd," added Ed.
7. The fan is fine and the bike is back, but I might have mice on the mat.
8. I shot a shout at the scouts and spotted Don downtown near the pond by the pound.
9. I fled the flood, but I bet a ton on number ten. I must have messed a bunch of stuff.
10. The fur is far from firm on the farm. I hurt my heart when I heard a hard sound.
11. There are points and pints of oil in the aisle. They tied the toys to the tiles.
12. The port is part of the court and the star is part of the store.
13. There's a hole in the hall and a ball in the bowl.
14. I pulled the fool from the pool and looked at Luke who stood in the stew.

# 7-2

# Vowel Slots Worksheet

Identify which vowel sound represents the highlighted letters in each word below. Use the key words at the bottom to help you decide.

| | | |
|---|---|---|
| 1. mix | 13. receipt | 25. cow |
| 2. house | 14. steak | 26. car |
| 3. height | 15. friend | 27. kind |
| 4. put | 16. pretty | 28. foot |
| 5. know | 17. season | 29. fruit |
| 6. apple | 18. hot | 30. says |
| 7. busy | 19. man | 31. ax |
| 8. hour | 20. men | 32. dough |
| 9. would | 21. women | 33. eye |
| 10. shoe | 22. does | 34. rain |
| 11. fall | 23. sew | 35. country |
| 12. cut | 24. crew | 36. able |

| i | ɪ | ɛ | æ | ɑ | ʊ |
|---|---|---|---|---|---|
| beat | bit | bet | bat | bought | book |

| u | ə/ʌ | eɪ | oʊ | aɪ | aʊ |
|---|---|---|---|---|---|
| boot | but | bait | boat | bite | bout |

# 7-3

# Minimal Pairs Diagnostic Worksheet: Vowels

| # | A | B | Contrast |
|---|---|---|---|
| 1 | fit | feet | /ɪ/ /i/ |
| 2 | bid | bead | |
| 3 | sin | scene | |
| 4 | gun | gone | /ʌ/ /ɑ/ |
| 5 | bum | bomb | |
| 6 | cup | cop | |
| 7 | set | sat | /ɛ/ /æ/ |
| 8 | blend | bland | |
| 9 | said | sad | |
| 10 | did | dead | /ɪ/ /ɛ/ |
| 11 | bit | bet | |
| 12 | disk | desk | |
| 13 | mate | mat | /eɪ/ /æ/ |
| 14 | main | man | |
| 15 | rake | rack | |
| 16 | cost | coast | /ɑ/ /oʊ/ |
| 17 | not | note | |
| 18 | want | won't | |
| 19 | buck | book | /ʌ/ /ʊ/ |

| 20 | putt   | put   |              |
|----|--------|-------|--------------|
| 21 | luck   | look  |              |
| 22 | fun    | fern  | /ʌ/ /ɝ/      |
| 23 | bud    | bird  |              |
| 24 | gull   | girl  |              |
| 25 | should | shoed | /ʊ/ /u/      |
| 26 | could  | cooed |              |
| 27 | look   | Luke  |              |
| 28 | dumb   | dome  | /ʌ/ /oʊ/     |
| 29 | rub    | robe  |              |
| 30 | fun    | phone |              |
| 31 | met    | mate  | /ɛ/ /eɪ/     |
| 32 | wet    | wait  |              |
| 33 | men    | main  |              |
| 34 | bowl   | boil  | /oʊ/ /ɔɪ/    |
| 35 | old    | oiled |              |
| 36 | tow    | toy   |              |

# 7-4

# /i/ vs. /ɪ/ Minimal Pairs Worksheet

|   | /i/ tense | /ɪ/ lax |
|---|-----------|---------|
| 1 | beat | bit |
| 2 | seat | sit |
| 3 | reed | rid |
| 4 | reach | rich |
| 5 | gene | gin |
| 6 | scene | sin |
| 7 | leak | lick |
| 8 | feast | fist |
| 9 | eat | it |
| 10 | steal | still |
| 11 | bean | bin |
| 12 | cheap | chip |
| 13 | peel | pill |
| 14 | leap | lip |
| 15 | green | grin |

## /i/ vs. /ɪ/ contrast sentences

|    | **/i/ (tense)** | **/ɪ/ (lax)** |
|----|-----------------|---------------|
| 1  | The dog beat him. | The dog bit him. |
| 2  | I'm sure my son won't sleep today. | I'm sure my son won't slip today. |
| 3  | That peach was perfect. | That pitch was perfect. |
| 4  | They didn't leave there. | They didn't live there. |
| 5  | She walks on heels. | She walks on hills. |
| 6  | She heats her rugs to clean them. | She hits her rugs to clean them. |
| 7  | Is that a big peak? | Is that a big pick? |
| 8  | He dropped the peel. | He dropped the pill. |
| 9  | Give me the meat. | Give me the mitt. |
| 10 | The week was very long. | The wick was very long. |

# 7–5

# Worksheet /ɛ/ vs. /æ/

|    | a. /ɛ/ | b. /æ/ |
|----|--------|--------|
| 1  | bend   | band   |
| 2  | Ken    | can    |
| 3  | set    | sat    |
| 4  | vest   | vast   |
| 5  | left   | laughed|
| 6  | sect   | sacked |
| 7  | send   | sand   |
| 8  | bed    | bad    |
| 9  | bet    | bat    |
| 10 | lend   | land   |
| 11 | met    | mat    |
| 12 | led    | lad    |
| 13 | tech   | tack   |
| 14 | rent   | rant   |
| 15 | blend  | bland  |

## /ɛ/ vs. /æ/ sentences

|  | **a.** /ɛ/ | **b.** /æ/ |
|---|---|---|
| 1 | Did you hear about the **bet** I made? | Did you hear about the **bat** I made? |
| 2 | I bought a **pen** yesterday. | I bought a **pan** yesterday. |
| 3 | Don't make a fuss about the **pest**. | Don't make a fuss about the **past**. |
| 4 | Did the **men** go to the game? | Did the **man** go to the game? |
| 5 | How come you couldn't see **any**? | How come you couldn't see **Annie**? |
| 6 | She **left** when he didn't come. | She **laughed** when he didn't come. |
| 7 | I don't want to **pet** the dog. | I don't want to **pat** the dog. |
| 8 | He'll **send** the furniture down. | He'll **sand** the furniture down. |
| 9 | I found the **kettle** in the barn. | I found the **cattle** in the barn. |
| 10 | What a **mess**! | What a **mass**! |
| 11 | Is it **dead**? | Is it **Dad**? |
| 12 | I **head** a team. | I **had** a team. |
| 13 | Where is the **vet**? | Where is the **vat**? |
| 14 | There are **ten** chairs over there. | There are **tan** chairs over there. |
| 15 | Is this the **men's** house? | Is this the **man's** house? |
| 16 | I didn't **peck** it. | I didn't **pack** it. |

# 7–6

# Vowel Contrast

### 3-way vowel contrast

|    | A. /æ/ | B. /ʌ/ | C. /ɑ/ |
|----|--------|--------|--------|
| 1  | cab    | cub    | cob    |
| 2  | bag    | bug    | bog    |
| 3  | sack   | suck   | sock   |
| 4  | stack  | stuck  | stock  |
| 5  | cap    | cup    | cop    |
| 6  | mask   | musk   | mosque |
| 7  | Dan    | done   | Don    |
| 8  | backs  | bucks  | box    |
| 9  | cat    | cut    | caught/cot |
| 10 | hat    | hut    | hot    |
| 11 | flax   | flux   | flocks |
| 12 | lack   | luck   | lock   |

## 3-way middle vowel contrast sentences

|   | A. /æ/ | B. /ʌ/ | C. /ɑ/ |
|---|--------|--------|--------|
| 1 | The caps are there. | The cups are there. | The cops are there. |
| 2 | The cat is on the rug. | The cut is on the rug. | The cot is on the rug. |
| 3 | Did you see the bag? | Did you see the bug? | Did you see the bog? |
| 4 | Is that Dan? | Is that done? | Is that Don? |
| 5 | I really hate gnats! | I really hate nuts! | I really hate knots! |
| 6 | It has to be last. | It has to be lust. | It has to be lost. |
| 7 | They stack it. | They stuck it. | They stock it. |
| 8 | They showed me their backs. | They showed me their bucks. | They showed me their box. |
| 9 | Where is the mask? | Where is the musk? | Where is the mosque? |

## 4-way vowel contrast

|   | A. /ɛ/ | B. /æ/ | C. /ʌ/ | D. /ɑ/ |
|---|--------|--------|--------|--------|
| 1 | den | Dan | done | Don |
| 2 | net | gnat | nut | knot |
| 3 | flex | flax | flux | flocks |
| 4 | tech | tack | tuck | talk |
| 5 | pen | pan | pun | pawn |
| 6 | mesh | mash | mush | mosh |
| 7 | sex | sax | sucks | socks |
| 8 | beg | bag | bug | bog |
| 9 | pecks | packs | pucks | pox |
| 10 | wren | ran | run | Ron |

# Syllables and Stress

## The Syllable

### Building Blocks

The syllable serves as the building block of the suprasegmental level of speech, and non-native speakers can improve their naturalness and intelligibility by developing a good awareness of its role and structure in English. Two areas are important to consider when working with non-native speakers: syllable structure (because of its importance in contrastive analysis of phonotactics), and syllable count (because of its connection to the endings of English, and as a stepping stone to work with lexical stress). Before continuing, however, consider Peter Ladefoged's (2001, p. 226) statement that "although nearly everyone can identify syllables, almost nobody can define them." Though linguists continue to debate definitions and properties of syllables, we can easily rely on our intuitive sense of syllables to guide our clients.

### Syllable Structure

At any given stage in its development, each language has set rules defining what types of syllables can possibly exist. Although there are many ways to define this structure, the two most important features for our purposes are the possible shapes of each syllable, and which specific consonants and vowels can fit within that shape. The most basic syllable in English can consist of a single vowel, and this is symbolized in linguistics by the capital letter *V*. An example of this type of word would be eye /aɪ/ or *owe* /oʊ/. At the other end of the spectrum, English allows a maximum of three consonants before a vowel, and four following it, which would be symbolized by CCCVCCCC, and exemplified by the word *strengths* when pronounced as /stɹɛŋkθs/.

The rules of English are much more complex in terms of exactly which particular phonemes can fit in each slot, as will be touched on in the section on phonotactics, and Table 8–1 outlines the basic combinations allowed in our language.

While non-natives do not need any explicit awareness of this, it is important for clinicians to consider when looking for clients' error patterns. For example, Korean has a maximum syllable structure of CVC. The *World Atlas of Language Structures Online* (Dryer & Haspelmath, 2013) categorizes languages such as Korean as in the moderately complex syllable group, which represents the majority (at 56.5%) of the 486 languages analyzed in the survey. English, on the other hand is categorized as a language with complex

**Table 8–1.** Permissible English Syllable Patterns

| Pattern | Example | IPA |
|---------|---------|-----|
| V | owe | /oʊ/ |
| VC | eat | /it/ |
| VCC | eats | /its/ |
| VCCC | acts | /ækts/ |
| VCCCC | angst | /æŋkst/ |
| CV | see | /si/ |
| CVC | seat | /sit/ |
| CVCC | cats | /kæts/ |
| CVCCC | casts | /kæsts/ |
| CVCCCC | sixths | /sɪkθs/ |
| CCV | ski | /ski/ |
| CCVC | threat | /θɹɛt/ |
| CCVCC | threats | /θɹɛts/ |
| CCVCCC | stunts | /stʌnts/ |
| CCVCCCC | twelfths | /twɛlfθs/ |
| CCCV | stray | /stɹeɪ/ |
| CCCVC | street | /stɹit/ |
| CCCVCC | streets | /stɹits/ |
| CCCVCCC | splints | /splɪnts/ |
| CCCVCCCC | strengths | /stɹɛŋkθs/ |

syllable structure, as are about 30% of the world's languages. A quick glance at the allowable maximum syllable structure of a client's language is an easy way to gauge possible difficulties with English phonology. The maximum syllable structure of Hawaiian, for example, is CV, while for Russian, it is CCCCVCCCC. Since the allowable structures in English place it in the minority of world's language, we can expect many clients to have difficulties with the initial and final clusters in English words, and a quick comparison of possible syllable shapes provides some insights.

## Phonotactics

Another important parameter involves the specific types of consonants that can fit in a given slot, and this relates to phonotactics. Phonotactics are a language's rules governing the sequencing of phonemes. If we look at the maximum syllable structure of Spanish, it is CCVCC, but in the initial cluster, the first element can only be the phonemes /b,k,d,f,g,p,t/ and the second element can only be either /l/ or /r/. In Mandarin, there are no clusters, and the only word final consonants are /n,ŋ/. When we describe the maximum syllable structure of English simply as CCCVCCC, we are leaving out some details that may inform our work with non-native clients. If we look at the initial CCC, there are actually only a few possibilities that are common in English, as shown in Table 8–2.

The only other 3-element clusters allowed in English are /skl/, which is found in words such as *sclerosis* /sklɚoʊsəs/ and is rare, and /sfr-/ which is reserved for Greek loanwords such as *sphrigosis* /sfrɪʤoʊsɪs/ and is extremely uncommon. Here are some other examples of English phonotactics:

- English does not allow gemination, so lengthening of consonants is not phonemic as it is in languages such as Hungarian, where *megy* [mɛɟ], (goes) and *meggy* [mɛɟː] (sour cherry) are minimal pairs

- /ʒ, ŋ/ do not occur phonemically in initial position

- /h, j, w/ do not occur phonemically in final position

**Table 8–2.** Initial Three-Element Clusters in English

| Cluster | Word |
|---------|------|
| /spl-/ | splash |
| /spr-/ | spray |
| /str-/ | street |
| /skr-/ | screw |
| /skw-/ | square |

## Syllable Count

A third area our clients should develop awareness of is the number of syllables in a given word, and this is where the true connection to the larger suprasegmental features comes into play. English words can vary from one syllable (in a word like *house*) to potentially dozens (in chemical compound names), but the vast majority lie in the one to six range. Some agglutinative languages commonly feature long multisyllabic words; the word *mutatóujjaitokkal*, which means "with your index fingers" in Hungarian, is eight syllables long, but other languages, such as Vietnamese, are almost entirely monosyllabic. Clients whose native languages feature longer words are more likely to have awareness of how to reproduce the correct number of syllables for English words, in comparison to their colleagues whose L1s generally feature short words. Clients need to produce English words with the same number of syllables as native speakers do to be intelligible and natural, and a good awareness of syllable count also helps them develop an understanding of the rules for past tense and -*s* endings.

Native speakers of English are usually given formal instruction on how to count syllables in elementary school, which indicates that the ability to identify the number of syllables in a word is not an essential part of natural L1 phonology acquisition, which does not normally require explicit instruction. As a result, native speakers are often poor syllable counters, as exemplified by a fair number of my undergraduate phonetics students. Nevertheless, whether they count accurately or not, native speakers of English will pronounce the citation form of a word in their dialect with the same number of syllables virtually every time. Non-native speakers may also have had some instruction in how to count syllables, either as a part of their instruction about how their own language works, or when they learned English in school, but they may also struggle with this task. In contrast to native speakers, however, they may produce the citation form of a word with a different number of syllables than a typical native speaker. While it is highly unlikely that any speaker of English will ever have to explicitly state the number of syllables in a word, the ability to count is a useful way for clients to develop the awareness necessary to monitor and compare their own productions to native models.

Clinicians can elicit information about syllables to probe their clients' abilities to count them accurately. Linguists devote considerable time to creating frameworks for syllables and even debating their definition, but it is probably not necessary to go into a great deal of detail with clients. In most cases, syllables fall into the "know it when I hear it" category, and after some training, clients should be able to agree on the numbers. Once again, the most important issue is the reproduction of a natural and accurate version of the word, so clients should develop a big picture sense that a syllable represents a "beat," which will help them tie it to the rhythm of our language. There are several useful tips to help clients count syllables. First, they can tap a desk or clap their hands with each beat; physical activity tends to work well for this, and even counting out with fingers is a typical strategy. Second, clients can monitor their jaw, possibly by placing their hand under it, in order to feel the movement that occurs as they produce each syllable. Last, they can hum the word, as this often makes it easier to break it into parts and count them.

**Table 8–3.** Sample Syllable Matching Exercise

Place these words in the appropriate box: relaxed, laboratory, stretched, characters, investigation

| Number of Syllables | Word |
| --- | --- |
| 1 | |
| 2 | |
| 3 | |
| 4 | |
| 5 | |

Scaffolding can help clients develop awareness, and can be accomplished by limiting their choices. An example activity is simply sorting words into two or more categories: words with one syllable and those with two. Listening discrimination can also help; clients can listen to words and sort them into columns. Focusing on just one- or two-syllable words can provide additional support, and clinicians should give challenging words such as *strength* that may appear to have two or three syllables based on orthography, even though it has only one. You can also have clients match words to boxes representing the number of syllables, where there is only one correct answer for each number, as shown in Table 8–3.

If clients need less structure, they can simply review lists of words and count out the syllables, or alternatively, they can provide examples of words with a given number of syllables. The following are some listening exercises clients can use:

- Listen to two words and determine whether they have the same number of syllables

- Listen to several words and determine which ones have a certain number of syllables

- Listen to words to determine whether the clinician produced it with the correct number of syllables or not. (Note that some clinicians are averse to providing any incorrect models during sessions out of a fear that the client will misremember it as a correct production.)

- Listen to syllable "minimal pairs" in which words or phrases can be contrasted by their number of syllables (e.g., "stretched" vs. "stretch it"). Clients can sort these into columns based on number of syllables.

Appendix 8–1 contains samples of these last two types of activities. At all stages, clients should be reminded that the actual goal is not the correct tally, but rather developing the awareness to produce the words with the same number of syllables as native speakers.

## Syllables and Vowels

Clients should be taught that vowels are key to identifying syllables, and they can use their knowledge of vowels to focus on the accurate production of monosyllabic words. Clinicians can tie syllables into training on vowels by asking clients to identify vowel phonemes and then state the number of syllables in the word. This should also help them with the typical problem of adding extra syllables based on word spellings, which we discuss below. Inform clients about the syllabic consonants of English, which are usually /ɹ,l,n,m/. The /ɹ/ consonant sound is included in the list, but it is probably better to just treat this as the /ɚ/ vowel. Examples of words with these syllabic consonants, such as *bottle, listen,* and *rhythm,* help clients focus on natural sounding speech, and will help with production of more challenging words such as *certain* or *mountain.*

Vowel syncope refers to unstressed vowels which "disappear" from words. The word *chocolate* is a good example. Originally a Nahuatl word, *chocolate* spread throughout the world in the 17th century, and it is pronounced in many languages with a vowel where our English spelling has an *o* letter but no vowel sound. The rules governing when these vowels are dropped relate to the sonority sequencing principle, but it would not be a worthwhile investment of time to go into theory when working with clients on such vowels. Clients can develop some awareness of these patterns and then monitor native speakers' productions to see if they mirror their own. The words tend to fall into two categories. In some words, such as *business* or *chocolate* the missing vowel is unlikely to reappear in any normal use, while for other words, such as *camera* or *memory,* the vowel can come and go depending on the speaker and context. Clients will often overpronounce these words if they are influenced by the spelling, especially if they have a cognate in their native language. While this topic is extremely valuable for helping clients attain natural sounding speech, it is probably best saved for more advanced clients since it will not affect intelligibility and may be distracting. Appendix 8–2 offers more examples of vowel syncope.

# Syllables and Endings

## Non-Native Errors

A logical extension of work with syllables is to practice regular past tense and -*s* endings since errors related to the rules for adding syllables are highly noticeable in these contexts. Many non-native speakers might err in producing a word such as *loved* with two syllables instead of one, and a word like *needed* with one syllable instead of two, and native speakers will catch this immediately. Although intelligibility might not be affected, it will certainly sound unnatural and draw attention to the speaker, as well as running the risk of being perceived as a grammatical error, which may be weighed heavily against the speaker. On the spectrum of languages with inflections, English has relatively few, but they still affect intelligibility and naturalness. Fortunately, the rules for the formation of the simple past and s endings have the advantage of being 100% regular, and clients should be able to use them correctly after some awareness building and practice. Many clients are aware of the rules from their English language instruction and may simply need a refresher, while other clients may have only a vague idea of how these inflections work. Native speakers learn these rules implicitly as toddlers and are generally unaware of them as adults.

## Regular Past Tense -*ed*

Many common English verbs have irregular past tense forms, and their pronunciation is generally addressed during accent modification training if clients are unsure about how a particular form is pronounced. The past tense of all the other English verbs is formed by adding the letters *(e)d* to the infinitive, and the pronunciation of those forms falls into three categories, as shown in Table 8–4. The rule is simple: take the final phoneme of the infinitive form of any regular English verb and if the final sound is /t, d/, add a syllable plus the /ɪd/ ending. In all other cases, do not add a syllable and pronounce -*ed* as /d/ if the final sound is voiced, and /t/ if it is unvoiced. There are no exceptions to this rule and it is highly productive (e.g., *skyped, googled, unfriended*). Keep in mind that this rule only applies to the regular past tense; there are several adjectives that also have the -*ed* ending but are pronounced in a way that might make them appear to be verbs that do not fit the pattern. These adjectives fall into two categories depending on whether they add an extra syllable in violation of the rules above at all times (such as *wicked*) or as an alternate form (e.g., *legged* as /lɛgɪd/ or /lɛgd/).

The additional syllable added for words ending in /t,d/ is the most salient of the three endings, and native speakers notice it immediately, so if a client produces *loved* as /lʌvɪd/, it will almost certainly be intelligible but not natural. When clients do not add the syllable, they may be misunderstood, depending on the context, and conversational partners may interpret it as a grammatical error. If a non-native says, "I needed to buy a car," but does not add the extra syllable in *needed*, it may sound like a plan for the future as opposed to a statement about the past. The voicing assimilation for the other two rules is clearly less important, especially because it really only applies to the /t/; non-native speakers who do not apply this rule are likely to overapply -*ed* as /d/ and not /t/. Because

**Table 8–4.** Rules for Pronouncing the Regular Past Tense

| Final phoneme | Example | Ending | Syllable added? | Example |
|---|---|---|---|---|
| /t,d/ | need<br>/nid/ | /ɪd/ | Yes | needed<br>/nidɪd/ |
| Any voiced sound other than /d/ (including all vowels) | love<br>/lʌv/ | /d/ | No | loved<br>/lʌvd/ |
| Any unvoiced sound other than /t/ | laugh<br>/læf/ | /t/ | No | laughed<br>/læft/ |

of this, it is essential to monitor for any failures to apply the first rule because that merits direct training. If clients are able to apply the first rule (regarding the addition of a syllable) regularly, but not the other two, then this will be a lower priority to address.

Past tense words that are produced with an additional syllable also represent an opportunity to either introduce the alveolar tap or continue to develop awareness of it. When a word such as *chat* is produced in the past tense, the /t/ becomes intervocalic and is normally produced faster and without full closure, resulting in the form [ʧærɪd]. Clinicians can take advantage of the large number of taps that will result when practicing words which follow rule requiring the additional syllable.

To assess awareness of these rules, clinicians can simply ask clients if they are aware of them, since many clients will have learned them early in their English instruction. Clinicians can provide clients with examples of words featuring the three types of endings and ask for an explicit statement of the rule. Appendix 8–3 gives clients the opportunity to discover the rules on their own and practice its application. Once again, make sure clients understand when to add the additional syllable, and then decide whether it is worth developing awareness of the voicing assimilation. The application of these rules can be practiced through structured activities with feedback focused on accuracy, or with spontaneous speaking tasks designed to promote carryover.

## The -*s* Ending

The -*s* has five functions in English:

- to mark the third person present tense of verbs (*flies*)
- to mark the plural (*streets*)
- as the possessive (*the boy's shoe*)
- as a contraction of the verb *is* (*what's she doing*)
- as a contraction of the verb *has* (*she's been tired lately*)

Since the last two are contractions and not endings, the rules below do not apply. The rules for pronouncing the final -*s* are shown in Table 8–5.

**Table 8–5.** Rules for Pronouncing the *s* Ending

| Final phoneme | Example | Ending | Syllable added? | Example |
|---|---|---|---|---|
| /s,z,ʃ,ʒ,ʧ,ʤ/ | *judge* /ʤʌʤ/ | /ɪz/ | Yes | *judges* /ʤʌʤɪz/ |
| Any voiced sound other than /z,ʒ,ʤ/ (including all vowels) | *love* /lʌv/ | /z/ | No | *loves* /lʌvz/ |
| Any unvoiced sound other than /s,ʃ,ʧ/ | *laugh* /læf/ | /s/ | No | *laughed* /læfs/ |

To simplify these rules, just add a syllable for /s,z,ʃ,ʒ,ʧ,ʤ/and then in all other cases, assimilate the voicing of -*s* (either /s/ or /z/) to the final sound of the infinitive without adding a syllable. There are no exceptions to this rule and it is highly productive (e.g., *sporks, ubers, zhuzhes*).

Once again, of the three possible endings, the most salient type of error would be a failure to apply the first rule since the incorrect addition or omission of a syllable is noticed instantly and might lead to miscommunication. The voicing assimilation for the other two rules is even less important than it is for the -*ed* ending for two reasons. First, once again, the /s/ will probably be overapplied, but if it follows an unvoiced consonant, it will be accurate. Second, final /z/ phonemes are somewhat devoiced in final position in English, so it may be barely perceptible if a client substitutes an /s/. The syllable rule is clearly the most important, but based on experience with non-native clients, errors with this rule seems to be less common than the rule requiring an additional syllable for infinitives ending on /t,d/ for the regular past tense; clients more commonly to produce "loved" than "loves" with two syllables. On the other hand, it is much more common for clients to add extraneous -*s* endings in spontaneous speech or when reading texts. Clinicians tend to disregard these errors because they are so unexpected, but they should be addressed if they occur as a regular pattern. As with the -*ed* ending, training can progress from awareness activities and structured practice through spontaneous speech tasks. Appendix 8–4 offers an opportunity for clients to discover the rule and put it into practice.

# Lexical Stress

## English Stress

Perhaps the most important reason for promoting awareness in syllables is to lead into work related to lexical stress since stress plays a crucial role in both intelligibility and naturalness. Compare the English words *insight* and *incite*. Although one is Germanic and the other is Latin, and their meanings are entirely unrelated, a broad transcription of both words is identical: /ɪnsaɪt/. While they might appear to be homonyms, when the words are pronounced there is a clear difference between the two. *Insight* is pronounced with stress on the first syllable [ˈɪnsaɪt] while *incite* is pronounced with stress on the second syllable [ɪnˈsaɪt]. Although pairs such as these are relatively rare in English and almost never involve words representing the same part of speech, their mere existence makes English different from many of the world's languages. While non-native speakers may not need to worry about this relatively rare phenomenon, what is highly relevant for them is that in English, word stress plays a prominent role in producing clear and natural speech, but it is not entirely predictable. If clients put stress on the wrong syllable there is an increased chance of misunderstanding. Hahn (2004) conducted a study of non-native teaching assistants and found that correct primary stress placement resulted in higher listener ratings of the speakers, demonstrating "a clear impact on listeners' perceptions of a speaker's ability to communicate." (Hahn, 2004, p. 215)

The role of lexical stress in the world's languages exists along a continuum. In some languages, stress is absolutely fixed; in Hungarian, for example, every word is stressed on the first syllable regardless of word length or origin. Polish features penultimate stress, so the next-to-last syllable always receives stress. Languages such as Spanish have a set of typical rules, but there are many exceptions which are marked in orthography. At the other end of the spectrum are languages such as Russian, whose stress was described by a Russian friend as behaving like a drunken flea. English falls somewhere in the middle, so there are some typical patterns and regularities, but there are many words that defy expectations, and even native speakers may place stress on the wrong syllable of a word they have never heard pronounced.

Before moving on to the stress patterns of English, it is important to define stress in a way that is meaningful for our clients. There is a great deal of technical debate about what constitutes stress and how it is produced, and since it involves both production and perception, the precise mechanics can be difficult to unravel. Nevertheless, in terms of the big picture, stressed syllables jump out in comparison to their neighbors, so they are said to have prominence. Speakers expend energy to make these syllables more noticeable, and we can divide the factors that help them stand out in English into four parameters, the first three of which are used in various proportions to create stress in most languages, and the last of which applies to a smaller group of languages such as our own. The first three typical determiners are pitch, loudness, and length, with each language using a different combination of these factors. In English, there is no set formula, so we look at general patterns, but we tend to prioritize them in this order: length, pitch, and loudness. It is important to develop a good awareness of the role each of these factors plays to monitor clients who are favoring one of them unnaturally. For example, by practicing marking stress through predominantly focusing on saying syllables louder, you will notice that this differs from the typical way native speakers pronounce words. Clinicians should always monitor clients' stress through the lens of our own system of producing it and stay alert for anything that strays from American English patterns. For example, when the last syllable of a word is stressed, there is a pitch glide, but when other syllables are stressed, the pitch drops. Thus, if a client produces a word such as *reply* with a sharp drop instead of a glide at the end, it sounds unnatural.

Because each language produces stress in slightly different ways, non-native speakers need to focus not only on placing the stress on the correct syllable of English words, but also on producing that stress naturally. In comparison to many other languages, stressed syllables in English tend to sound more prominent. A visual representation of the way a native speaker of English says the name of the city Yokohama looks different from that of a native Japanese speaker:

| English | Japanese |
|---|---|
| Yo-ko-HA-ma | Yo-ko-HA-ma |

Although Japanese does place stress on syllables, it is less noticeable than in English, so when native speakers of Japanese speak in English, they often sound flatter, as if they are speaking in a monotone. This may even be one of the reasons we pronounce some Japanese words in two ways, e.g., *Hiroshima* as "HiroSHIma" or "HiROshima. It is harder for us to hear differences in Japanese stress so we may override it and produce the word in a way that would better fit patterns of English. Many languages spoken by our clients will produce stress in a way that differentiates it perceptually from English. As an example, Delattre (2009) compared syllable lengths in English, German, Spanish, and French, and showed that English and Spanish differed most significantly for ratios of stressed to unstressed syllables (3.339 to 1 and 1.77 to 1, respectively. When he analyzed differences in vowel intensity for stressed versus unstressed syllables, he found that average differences of 4.4 dB for English, 2.2 dB for German, and only 1.3 dB for Spanish.

The fourth and last parameter we use to alter stress, vowel quality, affects English, but not all languages. In English, vowels can change their quality depending on whether they are in a stressed syllable or not. The example of *insight* and *incite* were used above because a vowel quality effect is not noticeable in that pair. More frequently cited pairs used to demonstrate stress differences based on vowel quality are *dessert*/*desert* (n.) and *object* (n.)/*object* (v.), and in these examples we can see the effect of vowel quality by examining what happens to the unstressed vowel:

desert (n.) = [ˈdɛzɚt]

dessert = [dəˈzɝt]

object (n.) = [ˈɑbʤɛkt]

object (v.) = [əbˈʤɛkt]

In the first pair, the /ɛ/ became /ə/, and in the second pair the /ɑ/ became /ə/; thus, in both cases the clear vowels were reduced to a schwa when the stress shifted. In some languages, such as Spanish, the stress on a vowel can shift, but the vowel is never reduced, it is just unstressed. The /a/ in the Spanish word *árbol* is stressed and the word is pronounced /ˈarβol/, and if we add a diminutive ending it becomes /arβoˈlito/ and the stress shifts to the penult; the vowel, however, is still an /a/. In English, vowels are often reduced, and that adds an additional factor for our clients to consider. There is some evidence that vowel reduction may impact intelligibility even more than correct stress placement (Lepage & Busa, 2013), but from a clinical perspective, it is clear that both of these interconnected features should be targeted during training.

## Stress Patterns

Most discussions about placement of stress in English begin with two-syllable words since monosyllabic words do not offer a choice of syllables. Nevertheless, the point mentioned above about vowel quality still applies to one-syllable words in connected speech, which means that some words have two forms depending upon whether the word itself receives stress in a sentence or not. The citation word for the auxiliary verb *do* for example, might look like /du/, but if it does not receive stress in a sentence, it might be pronounced as /də/. English speakers are aware of these reductions, and when they want to make it clear that a speaker is using them they will sometimes write them in what is sometimes called "eye dialect," as in "whaddaya mean" for "what do you mean."

According to Teschner and Whitley (2004), 75% of ordinary prose consists of monosyllabic words, and 90% of prose comprises only mono-and bisyllabic words. Once we begin to examine words with two or more syllables, we must consider which syllable receives primary stress, as every English word, regardless of length, has one syllable that receives more stress than any other. If we were working with a language such as Hungarian or Polish where stress is predictable, we could explain stress rules very quickly, and if our students were acquiring Spanish, we could provide them with a few basic overarching rules, and then point out some exceptions and details as their proficiency increased. Given sufficient detail, the rules governing English stress can be explained, but that level of detail is hard for clinicians to justify when working with non-native speakers on accent modification. Entire books are written on the subject of English stress alone, but it is hard to imagine that non-native speakers would benefit from delving into this level of analysis. It is more productive for clinicians to provide some familiarity of the basic patterns of stress and then encourage a high level of awareness so that clients will be laser focused on anything that strays from these patterns.

The basic rules for English stress revolve around three main factors related to phonology, morphology, and syntax. There is a fourth factor related to word origin that may sometimes be helpful as well. The phonological factors involve the number of syllables and their shape, the morphological factors are mostly related to suffixes and prefixes, and the syntactic factor that is most important is word class.

A good starting point for building clients' awareness is to focus on two-syllable words since there are really only two patterns to learn. Practicing the two patterns with nonsense words, modeled by the clinician and repeated by the client, and using some kind of visual reference provides scaffolding for the client. Clinicians can draw images, such as the following, and then contrast DA da with da DA:

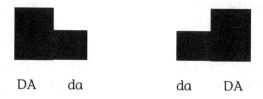

DA    da         da    DA

The actual shapes are not important as long as their relative size is indicated. The examples of unstressed vowels can be reduced since the client should focus on that effect as well. As a follow-up, clinicians can read lists of two-syllable words and have clients sort them into two categories, one category with the first syllable stressed, and the other with the second syllable stressed.

At this point, clients can begin to sort out how these patterns apply more broadly to English. Corpus studies have shown that nearly 75% of two-syllable words are trochaic

(Levis & Moyer, 2014), so clients are safest picking the first syllable to stress, but clinicians should point out the relationship between word class and stress in bisyllabic words. If clients are asked to list two-syllable nouns, they will produce words such as *water*, *apple*, *paper*, *bottle*, *teacher*, and if the clinician elicits the stress pattern for those words, the clients should quickly realize that most English two-syllable nouns are stressed on the first syllable. Clients often need some redirection if they are producing words that are not nouns or words that have more than two syllables, but if they produce two-syllable nouns, they are highly likely to name only those with stress on the first syllable since those vastly outnumber their counterparts with stress on the second syllable. To help them identify exceptions to this rule, clinicians can elicit 2-syllable nouns which are stressed on the second syllable. Clients will have to think carefully, but this kind of elicitation is a good opportunity for them to gain awareness of how to identify stress in a word. If they are unable to think of any examples, offer suggestions such as *hotel*, *police*, and *dessert*. Ask clients if they know that these words were originally French; most of the exceptions to the first-syllable stress pattern are words loaned from French to English. While we don't expect clients to have a well-developed sense of English etymology, their native language may have similar loan words from French so it worth a quick reference to this information.

The next step is to elicit two-syllable verbs. Clients should begin to list items like *deny*, *reply*, *attack*, *prepare*, which should lead them to notice that the predominant pattern for these words is to stress the second syllable. The majority of two-syllable verbs are stressed on the second syllable. This pattern is not quite as pervasive as the noun pattern (first syllable stress), so clients might list words such as *listen* or *worry*. If they do, ask them which pattern seems more common. While these exceptions stressed on the first syllable tend to be Germanic as opposed to Romance, there are so many exceptions that pointing this out may not help them.

It is a worthwhile investment to spend time working with clients on these basic two-syllable patterns before attacking longer words because many clients will still need to develop their skills, and with two-syllable words there are more regularities and only two possibilities. Once clients are confident with two-syllable nouns, the two-syllable verbs will require more effort since clients will encounter many more words that do not fit the expected pattern in comparison to nouns. Clinicians can use listening discrimination exercises by reading lists of verbs featuring both stress patterns and asking clients to identify which syllable is stressed. Clients can also read lists of two-syllable verbs and sort them into columns representing each stress pattern. Mazes are a fun and engaging way to provide clients with practice on making quick determinations of stress. Appendix 8–5 is a sample maze for adaptation or use. See *Pronunciation Games* by Mark Hancock (2012) for more maze ideas.

Stress patterns based on syntax apply to words that share the same form, and native speakers are aware of this phenomenon. There is a list of English oddities that sometimes makes the rounds, and one of the sentences on it is, "I did not object to the object." There are about 300 such noun/verb pairs from Latin that follow the pattern outlined above—the noun is stressed on the first syllable and the verb on the second. Native speakers themselves mix these patterns up when they are reading something aloud and need to make a quick decision based on context, but they usually stop and make a correction once they realize their mistake. Most clients are aware of this feature of English, but they often need practice on it, and it is a great opportunity to introduce the role of vowel reduction in shifting stress. Clients can be shown the basic pattern, which fortunately matches that of other English nouns and verbs, and then asked to identify what else happens when the stress changes. If they listen to the words *object* (n.) and *object* (v.), they should be able to point out that the /ɑ/ vowel sound found in the noun becomes /ə/ in the verb. Clients practicing these pairs should focus on both the stress pattern and the vowel reduction, and there are many practice activities that work well. Two typical activities involve sentences similar to the one described above ("I did not object to the object."), where clients read the sentence and produce the stress correctly on the noun and verb, or read sentences that feature either a noun or verb and decide which pattern to use. Appendix 8–6 includes examples of both activities. In the first type of activity clinicians can include spoilers which do not feature a stress shift, such as the word *surprise*, which comes from Latin but has stress on the second syllable for both the noun and the verb.

Numbers ending in *-ty* and *-teen* are also troublesome contrasts and allow clinicians to demonstrate examples of words whose stress patterns shift depending on context, such as *fifteen* and *fifty*. When said in isolation, clients should be able to hear that the word *fifteen* is stressed on the second syllable, while *fifty* has primary stress on the first syllable. Unfortunately, it is a little more complex when clients need to identify the stress patterns of these same two words in the following sentences:

I read fifteen pages of my book last night.

I read fifty pages of my book last night.

Clinicians can explain that the stress pattern is now identical since both words are stressed on the first syllable in this context. Give clients an opportunity to discover the rule on their own by trying to determine what happens in the following situations:

- fifteen
- I read fifteen pages of my book.
- I stopped reading at page fifteen.

With some guidance, they should identify that when the word *fifteen* is used attributively (i.e., before a noun), the stress shifts to the first syllable, but when it occurs in isolation or at the end of a phrase, the stress is on the second syllable. To help internalize this concept, ask the client to predict where the stress falls when native speakers are counting; they should realize that it shifts to the first syllable again when we count out "thirteen, fourteen, fifteen, sixteen. . ."

These rules apply to all of the *-teen* numbers, and clients should practice them since they are high frequency, either through minimal pairs or communicative activities, to ensure that they can generalize. On a side note, there is no reason to avoid discussion of the strategies native speakers use when they fear misunderstanding these numbers due to loud noise or other communicative factors. Many native speakers resort to questions such as, "Did you say five-oh, or one five?" to seek clarification, and clients should be armed with similar strategies to prevent communication breakdowns as long as they do not use them as a crutch. This is also a good time to practice other words that have stress shift when used attributively, as in the following example:

He speaks ChinESE.

The CHInese writing system is difficult to learn.

Consider the relative frequency of longer words before moving on to them. Of the 100 most common words in English cited in *The Reading Teacher's Book of Lists* (Kress & Fry, 2016), 94 are monosyllabic, and the rest are made up of two syllables. The frequency of words is directly related to their length, so while it is not unusual to hear words ranging from two to five syllables in conversation and more formal situations, words of six syllables and more are rare. Clients generally benefit most from focusing on words in the two- to three-syllable range first, since these are vastly more common in most communication, and later on words in the four to five syllable range. Understanding the relative frequency of stress patterns will also help clients essentially play the odds if they have some instruction on which stress patterns occur most often. A study conducted by Clopper (2002) looked at the frequency of all possible two to four-syllable stress patterns in English, and several of the results are informative for working with non-native clients. Two- and three-syllable words are more likely to be stressed on the first syllable than the second, but in four-syllable words, the second syllable (followed by the third syllable) is most commonly stressed. The rarest stress patterns are three- and four-syllable words stressed on their last syllable. A visual ranking of the frequencies from Clopper (2002) is shown in Table 8–6.

**Table 8–6.** Stress Frequencies Ranked (Clopper, 2002)

| Rank | Number of Syllables | Syllable Stressed | Example |
| --- | --- | --- | --- |
| 1 | 2 | 1st | water |
| 2 | 3 | 1st | activate |
| 3 | 2 | 2nd | attack |
| 4 | 3 | 2nd | atomic |
| 5 | 4 | 2nd | remarkable |
| 6 | 4 | 3rd | photographic |
| 7 | 4 | 1st | appetizer |
| 8 | 3 | 3rd | employee |
| 9 | 4 | 4th | Vietnamese |

Clients can gain awareness about stress for three- and four-syllable words by reviewing the possible patterns in Table 8–6. They should notice that the number of patterns is the same as the number of syllables, so there will be four possible ways to produce a four-syllable word. When working with longer words, clients should review the strategies they are using to determine which syllable is stressed. One strategy is to practice saying each longer word with stress on a different syllable to determine which one sounds best. For example, a client could produce *remarkable* as "REmarkable," "reMARKable," "remarkABle," and "remarkabLE." Another technique that is popular with my phonetics students is the "dog-calling" method in which clients can pretend to call a dog whose name is the same as the word. If we imagine calling out to a dog named "Remarkable," we would yell out "reMARK-able." Both of these techniques have the disadvantage of relying to some extent on feel, but by contrasting and exaggerating stressed syllables, the client may build awareness.

As clients begin to work on longer words, they may point out that they feel a certain amount of stress on more than one syllable of the word, which is a good opportunity for the clinician to review different levels of stress in English. There are many theoretical frameworks for analyzing these different levels of stress in English, but for practical purposes it is probably best to use a three-level system with clients consisting of strong, weak, and unstressed syllables. Strong syllables are those with primary stress, while weak syllables are those with secondary (or even tertiary) stress. In a word such as *academic*, there is weak (secondary) stress on the first syllable and strong (primary) stress on the third syllable. Note that weak stress is generally only noticeable in the citation form of a word. In comparison to work on primary stress and vowel reductions, secondary stress should always take a back seat since it is unlikely to significantly affect intelligibility or naturalness, especially in spontaneous continuous speech.

## Morphology and Stress

Up to this point we have analyzed stress in terms of phonology (how many syllables are in the word), syntax (i.e., whether the word is a noun or verb), and even word origin (French loan words tend to use an alternate stress pattern for two-syllable words), which leaves morphology as the final factor. When we add an affix to a word, the stress pattern can be affected. Once again, if we look for an easy way to apply a set of rules, we will be disappointed, but showing a few major patterns to clients helps them develop the awareness necessary to improve the accuracy of their lexical stress.

While there is no one overarching set of rules that explains what happens when affixes are added to words, we can break things down in several meaningful ways. If we approach it in a binary fashion, we can say that when an affix is added to a word it can either affect the stress of the word or not affect it. For example, the suffix *-ic* affects the stress of the original word, so if we add *-ic* to the root word *athlete* the stress will shift from the first syllable in *athlete* to the second syllable in *athletic*. On the other hand, if we add the suffix *-ness* to a word, there is no effect on stress, so *happy* is stressed on the first syllable, as is *happiness*. A ternary system has been proposed in which the affix is said to either shift the stress in the word, shift the stress to itself, or not shift the stress in the word. In this case, a suffix such as *-ee* would be separated out since when it is added to a word, it becomes the stressed syllable (e.g., *employ*, *employee*), but few affixes behave this way, so the binary system is more practical.

English has a large number of affixes, and in most cases it would not be worth the effort to analyze large numbers of them, but clients should be exposed to some of the more common prefixes and suffixes and given some practice in applying the stress patterns that come into play when they are used. One approach is to provide clients with a list of words with various affixes and have them sort the words into two categories based on whether the affix affects the original stress of the citation form of each word or not. An example might look like this:

| rhetorical | consistency | solidify | managerial | commitment | intensely |
| picturesque | happiness | ability | residency | motherless | beautiful |
| investigation | uniformity | willingness | powerless | preservation | Japanese |
| resourceful | government | substantial | immediately | | |

Clients should be able to sort them into the following two groups:

Change stress with affix = *-ion, -ial, -ese, -ity, -ical, -esque, -ify*

No change in stress with affix = *-ness, -cy, -ment, -ful, -less, -ly*

At this point, they can work with the clinician to identify the stress rules for the affixes that produce change. For example, the stress shifts to the syllable before the suffix *-ity*, but it shifts to the suffix itself in the case of *-esque*. Sometimes reference is made to shifting stress to the penult (second to last syllable) or antepenult (third to last syllable), but in most cases it is easier to simply identify the stressed syllable as coming immediately before the suffix, and this is easier for clients to remember. Clinicians can focus on suffixes that are more common and provide practice with examples. Teschner and Whitley (2004) report that the *-al, -ity, -tion,* and *-ic(s)* suffixes account for 90% of stress shifts resulting from the addition of suffixes. Prefixes applied to verbs do not generally affect stress, as in words like *increase* (v.), or *outperform*, but they will often receive stress when part of a noun, as in *increase* (n.) and *outlier*. Prefixes can receive contrastive stress as in the following example: "I wanted to INcrease the level of funding not DEcrease it"; it is usually better to address this aspect when working on emphasis.

## Compound Nouns and Descriptive Phrases

Another feature of English stress that can cause difficulties for non-native speakers is the difference between the patterns for compound nouns versus descriptive phrases. Consider the different ways *white house* is produced in the following sentences:

The president lives in the White House.

My friend lives in a white house.

**Table 8–7.** Compound Nouns versus Descriptive Phrases

|  | What does he teach? | Where is he from? |
| --- | --- | --- |
| He's an ENGLISH teacher. | English | ? |
| He's an English TEACHER. | ? | England |

In the first sentence, the stress is stronger on the first word of the pair, and in the second sentence it is on the second word. English has a tendency to put stress on the first element of a compound noun which has a nonliteral meaning, and on the second element of a descriptive phrase in which the words are not idiomatic. Compound nouns can be written in three different ways in English: as two words (light bulb), as one word (baseball), and as a hyphenated word (shrink-wrap). Sometimes two or more forms are accepted. There is a basic stress rule that applies to compound nouns—the first word receives more stress than the second. If the word has more than one syllable, then the stress will fall on the syllable that normally has primary stress. There are tendencies related to orthography: 90% of closed compound nouns (spelled as one word) place stress on the first element, but when compound nouns are hyphenated or spelled as two words, stress in on the first element only 55% of the time (Teschner & Whitley, 2004).

In some cases, the compound noun has less of an idiomatic meaning. Consider what happens when we stress either *English* or *teacher* in the phrase, "He's an English teacher," as shown in Table 8–7. When *English* receives the stress, we are identifying the subject taught, but when *teacher* is stressed, then the teacher's origin is implied. Another example is phrases ending with *problem* as in *math problem* or *financial problem*. The stress patterns for phrasal verbs and their related nouns are analogous, so we stress the preposition on the phrasal verb *pick up*, but the first syllable of *pickup* when we use it as a noun or adjective.

This feature of English merits some practice, but there are a few reasons to avoid placing too much focus on it. First, although there are some interesting contrastive pairs, such as *black bird* versus *blackbird*, they are relatively rare and unlikely to lead to a misunderstanding. If non-native speakers place stress incorrectly, it will certainly affect naturalness, but there is little chance of this being a common occurrence. In addition, there are dialectal or idiolectal differences for compound nouns such as *ice cream* and *cream cheese*. Finally, there are exceptions such as *black market* and *living wage*, where stress is on the second element despite idiomatic meanings. Clients should develop some awareness of this effect and work at internalizing patterns. If they have some exposure to the concept and learn the overarching rule that stress is on the first syllable for these compounds, they will be able to watch for exceptions.

In the end, it is helpful when clinicians provide clients with a set of general rules to help them make educated guesses and create a framework for identifying irregularities. A set of rules that can be practiced might look something like this:

Rule 1: two-syllable nouns and adjectives tend to be stressed on the first syllable.

Rule 2: two-syllable verbs and prepositions tend to be stressed on the second syllable.

Rule 3: Compound nouns tend to be stressed on the first element, especially when spelled as one word.

Rule 4: Words with suffixes such as *-ical, -ial, -ity, -tion -sion, -logy,* and *-ify*, have stress on the syllable right before the suffix.

Rule 5: Suffixes such as *-ness, -ment, -er -or, -less, -ly, -ship, - hood, -ful,* and *-ize* do not affect stress.

Rule 6: A handful of suffixes take stress themselves, such as *-ee, -ese, -eer, -esque*.

# References

Clopper, C. G. (2002). Frequency of stress patterns in English: A computational analysis. *IULC Working Papers Online*, pp. 1–9. Retrieved from: https://www.semanticscholar.org/paper/Frequency-of-Stress-Patterns-in-English-%3A-A-Clopper/3404d56321a167b484a3daa0654ece56aa1b8aff

Delattre, P. (2009). A comparison of syllable length conditioning among languages. *International Review of Applied Linguistics in Language Teaching, 4*(1-4), 183–198.

Dryer, M. S., & Haspelmath, M. (eds.) 2013. *The World Atlas of Language Structures Online.* Leipzig: Max Planck Institute for Evolutionary Anthropology. Retrieved from http://wals.info on 2018-12-06.

Field, J. (2005). Intelligibility and the listener: The role of lexical stress. *TESOL Quarterly,* 39(3) 399–423.

Hahn, L. (2004). Primary stress and intelligibility: Research to motivate the teaching of suprasegmentals. *TESOL Quarterly,* 38(2) 201–223.

Hancock, M. (2012). *Pronunciation games.* Cambridge, UK: Cambridge University Press.

Harley, H. (2006). *English words: A linguistic introduction.* Oxford, UK: Blackwell Publishing Ltd.

Kress, J. E., & Fry, E. (2016). *The reading teacher's book of lists.*

Ladefoged, P. (2001). *A course in phonetics.* Boston: Heinle & Heinle, Thomson Learning.

Lepage, A., & Busa, M. G. (2013). Intelligibility of English L2: The effects of incorrect word stress placement and incorrect vowel reduction in the speech of French and Italian learners of English [Conference paper]. *Concordia Working Papers in Applied Linguistics, 5,* 387–400.

Levis, J. M., & Moyer, A. (2014). *Social dynamics in second language accent.* Boston, MA: Walter de Gruyter.

Teschner, R. V., & Whitley, M. S. (2004). *Pronouncing English: A stress-based approach.* Washington, D.C.: Georgetown University Press.

# 8-1

# Sample Syllable Practice Worksheet

**Counting Syllables: Listening**

Listen to the following words and decide if they sound natural. Do they have the right number of syllables? Mark them with a check (✓) or a cross (x):

1. crashed
2. strengthen
3. chocolate
4. exhibits
5. bandage

6. divorced
7. businesses
8. clothes
9. examination
10. necessary

| | More syllables | Fewer syllables |
|---|---|---|
| 1 | Hungary | hungry |
| 2 | police | please |
| 3 | stretch it | stretched |
| 4 | idea | I.D. |
| 5 | notice | notes |
| 6 | use it to sing | used to sing |
| 7 | is cool | school |
| 8 | decided | decide |

# 8-2

# Dropped Syllables

In each of the following words a syllable may be dropped. Put a line through the letter for the vowel that is not pronounced:

Example: business

1. chocolate
2. aspirin
3. favorite
4. vegetables
5. interested
6. awfully
7. physically
8. Catholic
9. camera
10. evening
11. practically
12. temperature
13. family
14. average
15. Wednesday
16. basically

# 8-3

# Sample Past Tense Worksheet

Compare these regular verbs and their past tense forms. Decide if you add a syllable in the past tense:

|   | Verb | Past Tense | Extra syllable? |
|---|------|-----------|-----------------|
| 1 | relax | relaxed | |
| 2 | need | needed | |
| 3 | assert | asserted | |
| 4 | smoke | smoked | |
| 5 | rearrange | rearranged | |
| 6 | decide | decided | |
| 7 | anticipate | anticipated | |
| 8 | punish | punished | |
| 9 | reelect | reelected | |
| 10 | attach | attached | |

You only need to add a syllable if the verb ends in one of two sounds. Look at the table and complete the rule:

---

**Regular Past Tense:** Add a syllable in the past tense when you add -ed to verbs ending in / / or / /. If the last sound is voiced, add /d/. If unvoiced, add /t/.

---

| Infinitive | Regular Past | /ɪd/ + syllable, /d/, or /t/? |
|---|---|---|
| chop | chopped | |
| massage | massaged | |
| wash | washed | |
| collide | collided | |
| buzz | buzzed | |
| change | changed | |
| relax | relaxed | |
| hurl | hurled | |
| commit | committed | |
| organize | organized | |
| hatch | hatched | |
| calculate | calculated | |
| screech | screeched | |
| remain | remained | |
| cough | coughed | |

# 8-4

# Sample -s Endings Worksheet

Compare these words with their -s forms. Decide if you add an extra syllable:

| | Word | -s Form | Extra syllable? |
|---|---|---|---|
| 1 | relax | relaxes | |
| 2 | splash | splashes | |
| 3 | eliminate | eliminates | |
| 4 | allow | allows | |
| 5 | world | worlds | |
| 6 | arrange | arranges | |
| 7 | pineapple | pineapples | |
| 8 | attack | attacks | |
| 9 | attach | attaches | |
| 10 | massage | massages | |
| 11 | assassination | assassinations | |
| 12 | sneeze | sneezes | |

You only need to add a syllable if the verb ends in one of six sounds. Look at the table and complete the rule:

**Final "s"**: Add a syllable when you add an -s to words ending in the following sounds: / /, / /, / /, / /, / /, / /.

Read each word aloud after adding an *-s* ending to each. Remember to add a syllable only when necessary:

1. lemon
2. office
3. rash
4. phase
5. graph
6. garage
7. attach
8. skirt
9. cloth
10. badge

# 8-5

# Stress Maze

Move from start to finish by connecting squares that have words stressed on the FIRST syllable:

| | | | | |
|---|---|---|---|---|
| Start Here | panache | foretell | portray | deny |
| panic | attic | alleviate | relate | accept |
| fallacious | ratify | arduous | adulation | monstrosity |
| repel | aghast | appetizer | cannibalize | religion |
| accentuate | allege | excusal | photograph | biography |
| deliver | alibi | radish | mechanism | dedication |
| correct | arrogant | allocate | arrange | corrupt |
| outlast | outcome | granular | fortify | End Here |

# 8-6

# Nouns and Verbs with Different Stress Patterns

**Practice 1**
Take turns reading the following sentences being careful to use the right stress pattern. Watch for vowel reductions:

1. You need to **insert** a paragraph here on this newspaper **insert**.
2. How can you **object** to this **object**?
3. I'd like to **present** you with this **present**.
4. The manufacturer couldn't **recall** if there'd been a **recall**.
5. The religious **convert** wanted to **convert** the world.
6. The political **rebels** wanted to **rebel** against the world.
7. The mogul wanted to **record** a new **record** for his latest artist.
8. If you **perfect** your intonation your accent will be **perfect**.
9. Due to the drought, the fields didn't **produce** much **produce** this year.
10. Unfortunately, City Hall wouldn't **permit** them to get a **permit**.

**Practice 2**
Take turns reading the following sentences being careful to use the right stress pattern:

1. He wanted to subject him to a horrible experiment.
2. I didn't want to insult him by publishing that nasty comment.
3. If you contract a disease, you should see a health care professional.
4. Although he made some improvement, he didn't progress enough.
5. You should behave better if you want to get out on good conduct.

6.  He wanted to desert the army and flee the country.
7.  There was a defect in the engine of the car he bought.
8.  He couldn't understand what he read in the digest.
9.  She found him an escort because he didn't want to go alone.
10. My schedule conflict is going to create a problem.

# Prosody

## Phrasal Stress

### Language Rhythm

We begin to learn the rhythm of our native language in the womb and because it is such a natural part of the way we speak, we never give conscious thought to what makes it unique. Non-native speakers use different rhythms which set their speech apart from the pulse of other languages. Most adults learning a second language do not focus on rhythm when they communicate, and if they do, they may be uncertain about how to adapt theirs to that of American English. This is rarely something addressed in language classes or texts, and native speakers are at a loss to help. Moreover, in the history of pronunciation pedagogy, there are some outdated concepts that persist despite the evidence against them. Fortunately, SLPs are attuned to the rhythms of language and can provide excellent modeling and coaching once they step back to consider how English works.

### Syllable Based Versus Stress Based

Intuitively, we know that the rhythm of English sounds different when spoken by native speakers as opposed to those learning English as a second language, and in the early years of the last century, pioneers in the world of accent began to theorize exactly where the distinction lay. The most significant development in this respect was in the 1940s, when Pike (1945) promulgated the idea that English is a "stress-timed" language, while many other languages are what he labeled "syllable-timed." There are several principles to the theory, but the basic idea is that there are two types of languages in the world, those in which the timing is equal between stress points, and those in which it is equal between syllables. This theory was designed to explain why certain words jump out at us in English, but when we hear a language like Spanish spoken rapidly, it has a staccato effect without the peaks we are accustomed to. One of Pike's greatest contributions was the idea of stress suppression to explain how certain words in English seem to be swallowed in speech. Since then, a great deal of evidence has accumulated disproving the assertions that objective measures can divide languages into these two timing-based categories, and the terms syllable-timed and stress-timed have been replaced with "syllable-based" and "stress-based." While researchers continue to learn more and more about the intricacies of rhythm, one unfortunate side effect of Pike's original formulation was his influence on TESOL pedagogy and accent instruction. One of the most popular pronunciation texts of the last century, *Manual of American English Pronunciation* was an adaptation of Pike's ideas, written by Clifford Prator in 1972. Wayne Dickerson of the University of Illinois has analyzed Prator's adaptation of Pike's ideas as well as his role in shaping the thoughts of the EFL teaching community since the 1950s. Prator and Robinett's book has several diagrams designed to illustrate the differences between English rhythm and that of other languages. While the English diagrams show families with some adults and some children to represent the fact that some words stand out due to their stress, the diagrams representing other languages show soldiers of uniform height. Over the years, various pronunciation texts have adopted analogies of this type, although they have used different imagery, such as busses and cars. Prator and Robinett were following Pike's lead in trying to develop a framework to explain how English stress is perceived by listeners, but as Dickerson (2015) points out, their main flaw was that they overapplied the amount of stress points non-native speakers should focus on. Possibly in an effort to simplify things, he advocated stressing content words, but instead, native speakers choose one or two stress points in each phrase and suppress the stress of most of the other words (including content words) in the phrase.

To understand how we can best help non-native speakers acquire the rhythm of English, we have to consider why so much research has gone into attempting to identify differences in stress patterns between languages, and why so many pronunciation textbooks have focused on rhythm. The answer is that we know intuitively that English sounds different, and once we have a look at some of the features that create this perception, we can guide clients to develop the awareness they need to shape their speech. The key is to have clients concentrate on just one or two stress points per phrase, and suppress the stress on the other words.

## Content Words Versus Function Words

A good starting point to understand why English is perceived to have such a different rhythm from other languages is to separate function words from content words and examine their role in connected speech. Content words are sometimes called "open class" words because new ones can be created at any time. We can consider these the software of language because new versions come out frequently, and to continue with the tech analogy, consider words such as *google, skype, landline* that have been added to the language in the recent past. Content words are mainly nouns, adjectives, adverbs, and adjectives. Function words are referred to as "closed class" words because they are more like hard-

**Table 9–1.** Content Words and Function Words

| Content Words | Function Words |
|---|---|
| Nouns (tree, house, John) | Pronouns (he, she, it) |
| Verbs (walk, run, read) | Articles (an, a, the) |
| Adjectives (yellow, big, five) | Prepositions (in, on, through) |
| Adverbs (happily, quickly, fast) | Quantifiers (a few, several) |
| | Conjunctions (and, or, but) |

ware—they may change, but not as often. Function words, such as articles, prepositions, and pronouns hold the language together. The last pronoun added to English was the word *she* over 1,000 years ago. Table 9–1 outlines the division between content and function words for clients, and clinicians can elicit a few more examples of each word class to ensure that clients are aware of the distinctions.

Verbs can be thorny because the parts that make up a verb form, such as the continuous form, fall into both content and function word categories. In the sentence, "He is reading," *is* is considered a function word and *reading* is the content word. Auxiliaries and modals fall into the function word category, even though they are verbs. Since the verb *have* is both an auxiliary and a regular verb, it can be stressed depending on the role it plays:

*Have* as a content word: "I have a nice house."
*Have* as a function word: "I have been there three times."

The verb *do* is also both an auxiliary and a regular verb, and we will look at how it affects stress as an auxiliary later, in the discussion on emphasis.

The difference in possible stress patterns is obvious when we compare the function words to content words because even though many of the function words are monosyllabic, they feature reduced vowels when they are unstressed. Consider the words in Table 9–2. If we ask native speakers to produce the words in isolation, we will get the citation form, but if we listen to the same words in connected speech, they will sound different.

The first step in achieving English rhythm is to destress these function words, and the ability to reduce the vowel gives clients an easy starting point to create more natural sounding speech, even if they still place too much energy on the words themselves. As an example, compare how the following words sound when read aloud:

*restaurant, for, went, dinner, the, I, to*
Compared to: "I went to the restaurant for dinner."

In the first version, the function words *for* and *to* would likely have clear vowels, and the word *the* might even be pronounced /ði/ in this context. When the function words are produced normally in a sentence, the vowels are reduced. Now say the second sentence but pronounce each word as if it were being pronounced in citation form. The sentence now

**Table 9–2.** Citation and Reduced Forms of Function Words

| Function Word | Citation Form | Reduced Form(s) |
|---|---|---|
| to | [tu] | [tə] |
| for | [fɔɚ] | [fɚ] |
| have | [hæv] | [əv] [ə]* |
| can | [kæn] | [kən] [kɪn] [kn̩] |
| and | [ænd] | [ən] [n̩] |
| or | [ɔɚ] | [ɚ] |
| of | [ʌv] | [ə] |
| do | [du] | [də]* |
| your | [jɔɚ] | [jɚ] |
| you | [ju] | [jə] |
| him | [hɪm] | [ɪm] |

*when auxiliary verb, not when regular verb.

sounds robotic and unnatural, and even though it is an exaggeration, it sound in some ways like the rhythm of some non-native speakers. Therefore, clients who use unnatural English rhythm should start with the mechanics of reducing vowels in the function words, and then practice destressing them as much as possible. Speakers of some languages with rhythms similar to English, such as Russian or German, will have no problem with this type of exercise, but other clients may struggle to distribute the stress unevenly as we do in English. There are about 40 common function words that feature vowel reductions, and clients should practice destressing them in sentences. During this phase of rhythm work, we can place some stress on content words, but in the end, many of those should be destressed as well, as we will see below. One typical method of acquiring destressing skills is to have clients practice saying sentences with the same number of content words, adding more and more function words to the sentence. For example, clients can say the sequence of sentences below, clapping out the stress on the content words, keeping it the same across all sentences:

> HELP MAKE LUNCH
> I'll HELP MAKE LUNCH
> I'll HELP MAKE his LUNCH
> I'll HELP you MAKE his LUNCH
> I can HELP you MAKE his LUNCH
> I can HELP you MAKE him his LUNCH
> I'd like to HELP you MAKE him his LUNCH

The key to this type of exercise is to have clients clap and keep the time between beats exactly the same for all of the sentences, which forces them to destress the function words.

Clients should always understand that in reality, these sentences will get slightly longer each time, and that we are artificially keeping the length the same as a way to practice destressing. They should understand, however, that we do not lengthen these sentences (with regard to the time it takes to read them) in proportion to the number of syllables added, so while "Help make lunch" has three syllables, "I'd like to help you make him his lunch" has nine. If we compare the length of time it takes to say each sentence naturally, the second one would be longer, but it would not be three times longer. If clients can compare what the second sentence sounds like three times longer, they will hear how unnatural stressing all of the words in a sentence sounds in English.

While the first step is the reduction of function words, the next step is to suppress the stress of some of the content words. As outlined above, one of the misconceptions about the rhythm of English is that content words should all receive stress. While stressing all of the content words in the sentence definitely sounds more like English rhythm compared to stressing all of the words in the sentence, it still sounds somewhat choppy. In the sentence, "I like to drink red wine," there are four content words: *like*, *drink*, *red*, and *wine*. Try saying the sentence with stress on all of the content words, but with *I* and *to* destressed and the vowel in *to* reduced, as in "I LIKE to DRINK RED WINE." Even if we jump up a little bit on the final content word (wine) to set it apart, the sentence sounds unnatural. The reality is that we generally pick one or two words to stress, depending on how we break it up into phrases, and all of the other words (including other content words) are destressed. The suppression of the stress on the content words might be less noticeable because the vowels inside the words will not be reduced. To summarize, in order to produce natural sounding English rhythm in connected speech clients should concentrate on the following:

1. Reduce vowels of the function words whenever possible, and destress them
2. Pick one content word as the focus of each phrase and give it the most stress
3. Reduce the stress on most (or all) of the other content words in the phrase

These guidelines will help clients develop their awareness, but ultimately, they need to develop a good sense of how to combine all of the suprasegmental-level parameters, including rate, intonation, and linking, to speak clearly and naturally. The question of which content words should receive stress can be tricky. Phrases typically have at least one content word that receives less stress than the focus word, and clients can practice destressing those words after they have a good sense of how to choose the focus word.

## Tonic Stress

Since we have discussed the importance of suppressing the stress on most of the words in a phrase, we now turn to selecting the element that should receive the most stress—the focus word—which receives what is called "tonic stress." This selected word is normally the last content word in a phrase, but depending on the context, a different word can be stressed, and we can call stressing that word "emphasis."

The focus word is the one word in each phrase that a speaker wants to stand out from those around it, so it mirrors the syllable with primary stress in a multisyllabic word. Stress is applied in the same way as with multisyllabic words: we make the word longer, higher, and louder to give it prominence. It is normally not at the highest pitch point in the sentence because pitch drops throughout the production of the utterance, but it stands out because of how it sounds relative to the other words in the phrase. In theory, stress can fall on any word in a sentence depending on context, but in most cases, the basic rule to determine which word is the focus word is that it's the last content word in a phrase. If we say the short sentence, "I went to the store," as one phrase, then the focus word would normally be *store*. While this rule provides a nice overarching framework, there are a couple of small points to consider. If other function words follow, they will normally not be the focus, so in the sentence, "I went to the store with him," *store* is still the focus word. If we add an adverb of place or time, unlike in other languages, English does not stress the adverb. So if we have, "I went to the store there," we would not make *there* the focus word, even though many of our clients might. If the last content word is a compound noun, the stressed element is the focus word even if it is the first element. So in the sentence, "I went to the grocery store," focus would be on *grocery* since it is the stressed word in the compound noun *grocery store*. Clients and clinicians should always keep in mind that selection of the focus word is entirely dependent on the context, so these examples are just typical tendencies. It will also depend on how the phrases are divided, so if we pause between *went* and *to*, as in, "I went/to the store," then both *went* and *store* would be the focus of their respective phrases.

As a final important note, the third rule above stated that most (or all) of the phrase's other content words should be destressed, but in a sentence such as, "I went to the store," there may be some additional stress on went. Clients will nevertheless benefit most by keeping their attention on the focus word, and then working to develop a sense of which additional words in a phrase can be given some additional stress. In longer phrases, clients need to be careful to avoid stressing too many content words or they will sound choppy, so concentrating on one focus word is usually the key to success.

## Reducing Modals and Auxiliaries

Reducing stress on modals and auxiliaries also makes clients sound more natural. They may find that producing phrases such as *could have gone* is difficult, especially if they are placing too much stress on the words. It is important to point out to them that auxiliaries such as *do* and *have* and modals such as *could* and *would* look like content words because they are verbs, but they are function words and can be reduced. Constructions such as *could have*, *would have*, and *should have* are extremely common, and English speakers sometimes use the expression "coulda, woulda, shoulda," which illustrates the reductions that take place when we produce these words. If a phrase ends with *have* we usually reduce the vowel but sometimes we keep the /v/. For example, the sentence, "I could have," sounds like either [aɪkʊrə] or [aɪkʊrəv], although in this context, the vowel in *have* could be /æ/. Clients should practice saying these forms in various ways to give

**Table 9–3.** Modal Reductions

| Modal + have | Clear | Natural | Example Sentence | Pronunciation |
|---|---|---|---|---|
| could have | [kʊdhæv] | [kʊrə] | I could have gone. | I "coulda" gone. [aɪkʊrəgɑn] |
| should have | [ʃʊdhæv] | [ʃʊrə] | I should have gone. | I "shoulda" gone. [aɪʃʊrəgɑn] |
| would have | [wʊdhæv] | [wʊrə] | I would have gone. | I "woulda" gone. [aɪwʊrəgɑn] |

**Table 9–4.** Reduced Forms of Can and Can't

|  | Citation Form | Reduced Form |
|---|---|---|
| can | [kæn] | [kən] [kɪn] [kn̩] |
| can't | [kænt] | [kænʔ] [kænt̚] |

them a feel for the natural speech continuum of informal to formal communication. Clients and clinicians tend to underestimate the amount of reduced speech that occurs in situations that might be considered formal, such as conference calls and presentations. Table 9–3 illustrates some of these forms.

Clients are bound to ask about the differences in how to pronounce the words *can* and *can't*, since these are often troublesome, and this is best addressed during a discussion of rhythm and vowel reduction. Many clients have had some experience with British English or other versions of English that feature distinct vowels for the citation form of these two modals, and they are confused about how Americans can tell them apart. If we look at the citation form of these words, we have /kæn/ and /kænt/; the only difference appears to be /t/, but when clients hear Americans saying these words, they notice that since we tend to not release the final /t/, the difference is minimal. There is, indeed, a difference between these two in terms of vowel length: native speakers lengthen the vowel for *can* and shorten it for *can't* because they still interpret the second word as having a /t/ even when they do not release it audibly. More importantly, however, is what happens to these words when they are in sentences. Table 9–4 shows the possible vowel reductions for the word *can*.

The final step is to show clients how these forms work in terms of English rhythm. The word *can* will be destressed and the stress tends to fall on the verb it is modifying, whereas *can't* used in a sentence usually receives some stress and retains its full vowel. Clients can benefit from drills on this concept to make sure that they do not produce the difference between these modals by just pronouncing the final /t/, or by simply overpronouncing to make the words clear. The main difference in pronunciation is based on how these words function in the rhythm of English.

# Emphasis

## Shifting Focus

One of the more challenging aspects of working on phrasal and tonic stress with clients is that stress patterns are highly dependent on context, and in theory it is possible for any word to become the focus of a phrase. When working with clients on the typical stress patterns of English, we might find that they produce a pattern that is possible in certain contexts. As an example, if a client is asked to read the sentence, "I saw the red car," we might expect stress to be placed on the last content word *car* because that is the standard pattern for a declarative sentence. Nevertheless, the client might produce the sentence with stress on *red*. Although we can correct the client and model the expected pattern, in reality, since there is no context, stress could be placed on any word in that sentence. If we consider the sentence as a response to two different questions, we can see that tonic stress can shift:

> What did you see? I saw the red CAR.
> Which car did you see? I saw the RED car.

This rhythm of English is so natural for native speakers that we tend to assume that non-native speakers will adapt to it easily, but that is not always the case, and this aspect of accent modification deserves attention when working to help our clients sound more natural.

There are several reasons English speakers shift the focus from the last content word in a phrase, which is the normal position for stress, and clinicians should walk clients through these functions to foster their awareness of them.

As demonstrated by the first example below, one of the most common reasons to shift emphasis is to answer a question appropriately. Look at the following exchanges:

> 1 A. Where did you go?
>    B. I went to the STORE.
> 2 A. Who went to the store?
>    B. I went to the STORE.

The context determines the appropriate emphasis, so while the first exchange would be considered typical, the second one sounds odd because the typical stress pattern for that sentence should place tonic stress on *I*. A second common reason to use emphasis is to correct information in response to either a question or a sentence:

> A. Are my socks on the CHAIR?
> B. No, they're UNDER the chair.

Or:

A. Santos Dumont invented the AIRPLANE.
B. No, the WRIGHT Brothers invented the airplane.

Note that the information provided does not actually have to be correct; the most important principle here is that the stressed word is the information that the speaker considers to be correct, independent of the focus word in the first statement or question. So in the first example the second speaker might respond with, "No, they're under the DESK." Emphasis is also used to highlight new information in response to a statement or question:

A. Dave is tired. / Is Dave tired?
B. Yes, he's VERY tired.

Or even when a single statement adds additional information, as in:

Dave is tired today. VERY tired.

As a variation of this principle, emphasis changes when a question or information is repeated, as in:

A. (to B) What did you think about the MOVIE?
B. It was great.
A. (to C) What did YOU think about the movie?
C. I didn't like it.

Or:

A. What did you think about the MOVIE?
B. I liked it. What did YOU think about it?

Emphasis can also highlight a contrast, as in:

She LIVES in Oakland, but she WORKS in San Francisco.

Note the double emphatic stress in this sentence because Oakland would normally receive tonic stress in a declarative sentence. And emphasis can indicate excluding something, as in:

He loves classical MUSIC, but he HATES opera.

By examining the uses above, we can see that in theory, any word can be stressed in any sentence given the appropriate context. Consider the phrase, "I told him to bike to work," based on the following contexts and decide which word to stress:

**I** told him to bike to work. Meaning: Someone else didn't tell him.
I **told** him to bike to work. Meaning: I didn't ask him.
I told **him** to bike to work. Meaning: I didn't tell someone else.
I told him **to** bike to work. Meaning: He thought it would be a good idea not to bike to work.

> I told him to **bike** to work. Meaning: Not to drive to work.
> I told him to bike **to** work. Meaning: Not from work.
> I told him to bike to **work**. Meaning: Neutral, or to emphasize work as opposed to somewhere else.

Before delving into additional advanced functions of emphasis and how to train clients to use them accurately, we must point out the difficulties clients may have with this suprasegmental aspect of English. When reading through the above examples, they may appear to be something obvious or unnecessary to explain because it is such a natural part of the way we communicate. In other languages, however, there are entirely different ways of expressing emphasis, so many clients may have insufficient awareness of how emphasis functions in English. In case-based languages, such as German or Russian, word order is more fluid because declensions indicate the role of each word (e.g., subject, direct object, indirect object), and in these types of languages speakers can change the position of a word in a sentence to emphasize it. Therefore, a German speaker can say a sentence that translates directly into English as, "Karl gave I the book," to focus attention on Karl as the recipient as opposed to Frank. In English we cannot reverse the order of subjects and indirect objects, but we can use emphatic stress to say "I gave KARL the book" In languages such as Spanish and Portuguese that feature pronoun dropping, the pronoun can be inserted for emphasis. Thus, a Spanish speaker can say, "Te creo" (I believe you), or add a subject pronoun and say "Yo te creo" (I believe you) to emphasize that the speaker believes someone and others do not. In other languages, particles or other means can express these ideas. If clients' awareness of the intricacies of emphatic stress in English are limited, they need some exposure to examples and practice. In addition, there is a strong prosodic component to the way these sentences are produced, so most clients need to concentrate on natural intonation and phrasing to produce them well. On a positive note, emphasis is in some ways more concrete than other aspects of intonation, and many clients who are shy about making significant changes in prosody to convey their emotions are more likely to conceptually grasp the need to place focus on a particular word to answer a question or correct another speaker. For this reason, working on the mechanics of emphasis may provide an opening for working with clients who resist encouragement to use more dynamic intonation. Appendix 9–1 features an activity in which clients shift the emphasis to different words in sentences containing *too* or *either* depending on prompts read by a clinician. For example, clients might see the sentence, "He works with his sister too." If the prompt is, "He works with his brother," the reply would be "He works with his SISTER TOO," but if the prompt is, "He lives with his sister," then the correct response is, "He WORKS with his sister TOO." Relatively concrete activities like these are a good starting point for clients who are reluctant to alter their pitch patterns.

## Advanced Functions of Emphasis

We can think of the correcting function of emphasis as a form of disagreement, and alternatively, we can use emphasis to agree with another speaker. What sets this function apart is that it creates an interplay between pronunciation and syntax. While the exchange below is certainly natural:

1. A. He plays guitar well.
   B. You're right. He plays guitar well.

It is probably more common to hear something more along these lines:

2. A. He plays guitar well.
   B. You're right. He DOES play guitar well.

In this case, speaker B expresses agreement with speaker A by adding an auxiliary verb and placing stress on it. Using an auxiliary follows the same rule as when forming other sentences in English: *do/does/did* for all verbs with the exception of the verb *to be* and the modals (*could*, *should*, *would*, etc.). Here are examples of how this would work with those exceptions:

Example 1:

A. He should do it right away.
B. Yes, he SHOULD do it right away.

Example 2:

A. She's easy to work with.
B. Yes, she IS easy to work with.

Note that in the example featuring the verb *to be* it is more likely to use the full form of the verb as opposed to the contraction even though both are possible. The use of emphatic auxiliaries is very common among native English speakers but it is often overlooked by non-native speakers. In some cases this is because clients overgeneralize some of the corrections they may have received in early stages of English acquisition. A beginning student of English might produce a sentence such as, "Yesterday, I did go to the store," without putting stress on the word *did* as a grammatical mistake, and the teacher might provide the correct model of "Yesterday, I went to the store." Once non-native speakers develop awareness for emphatic auxiliaries they begin to notice how common they are in everyday speech and can be encouraged to produce them. Emphatic auxiliaries can also show contrast, as in the following sentence:

"He's short, but he DOES play basketball well."

Another advanced use of emphasis is altering the normal stress pattern of the citation form of a word to place contrastive stress on a prefix. The words *disadvantage* is normally stressed on the third syllable, but in the sentence, "The advantage of having a car is that it makes getting around easier, but the DISadvantage is that it pollutes," the stress shifts to the prefix. Table 9–5 lists some sample pairs illustrating possible stress shifts to the prefix.

It is also possible to place contrastive stress on the prefixes of two or more words, as in the quotation attributed to Thomas Edison: "Genius is one percent INspiration, ninety-nine

**Table 9–5.** Possible Prefix Stress Shifts

| possible | IMpossible |
| --- | --- |
| likely | UNlikely |
| nationalistic | ULTRAnationalistic |
| relevant | IRrelevant |
| normal | ABnormal |
| typical | Atypical |

percent PERspiration," or in the sentence "I know some people who are MONOlingual, but I also know others who are BIlingual, or even MULTIlingual.

## Training on Emphasis

Generally, clients quickly develop an understanding of the communicative value of emphatic stress after they are shown a few examples, making it an excellent starting point for clients who are resistant to developing more natural prosody. Clients can usually identify which word is emphasized when they hear native speakers, but if they cannot, then training can begin with some listening discrimination in which they are simply asked to identify which word in a sentence is being produced by the clinician with emphatic stress. Clients can be given prompts containing sentences such as, "My friend's daughter drives to work every Wednesday," and the clinician can emphasize various words in the sentence and have the client identify which word was stressed. Alternately, you can do this activity without showing prompts, and clients can repeat the stressed word. The next step before having clients practice producing emphatic stress themselves might be to have them look at sentences and then identify which word would be stressed in response to a variety of questions. If they see the sentence:

She's in the bathroom.

They can point to (or read out) the word *she* if asked "Who's in the bathroom?" *in* if asked "Is she outside the bathroom?" and *bathroom* if asked "Where is she?"

To practice disagreeing/correcting, clients can use activities in which they use emphatic stress to correct an incorrect statement they hear. If the client hears, "There are 30 days in January," they would say something along the lines of "No, I think there are thirty-ONE days in January." Clients should be encouraged to provide any alternative information even if they don't know the correct answer, although discussing the prompts can also provide some opportunities for naturalistic conversation. Similarly, clients can practice agreeing by listening to statements and concurring, keeping in mind that they should try to add an auxiliary whenever possible. This might also prompt some discussion about English grammar; a client might ask if, "Yes, he DID used to live in Mali," is a possible response to agree with the sentence "He used to live in Mali." and the clinician would answer that this would work well, and point out that *used* becomes *use* following *did*. Clients can practice adding new information by creating sentences from prompts, so if they see or hear *wine/red wine*, they can produce a sentence such as "I love wine, especially RED wine." Appendix 9–2 provides examples of these types of activities.

Once clients have a good grasp of some of the basic uses of emphatic stress, they can apply these principles to develop a more dynamic speaking style. Clinicians can have clients bring in typical work presentations they may give and then coach them on jumping up to different pitch levels to help them develop a more engaging speaking style.

# Phrasing

Much of the rhythm of English depends on how speakers break up their speech. We have seen how the choice of focus words depends on where pauses occur, but there are many other factors related to these pauses that need to be addressed with clients. To illustrate quickly, think of the following sentences:

Sara said, "Don was tired."
"Sara," said Don, "was tired."

The punctuation tells the story in the written word, but in speech, pauses provide most of the clues to the meaning. There will always be a connection to intonation and other suprasegmental features, but several aspects of English communication make sense to address by looking at phrasing. There have been many terms used to describe these chunks of speech, such as *thought groups*, *intonation groups*, and *breath groups*, to name a few, and clinicians are free to use whichever descriptive term they prefer. I refer to it as *phrasing* because it is simple and it works.

It is a good idea to bring up phrasing early in accent training because it is intertwined with so many aspects of connected speech, and it is especially important to discuss it when working on tonic stress, since clients need to understand the relationship between pauses and focus words. As an example, we can take a phrase from the diagnostic passage included in Chapter 3 and divide it in several ways, with slashes representing pauses to isolate the phrases, and bolding for focus words:

Although children can easily learn to speak a second language with a native **accent**,/ adults are not as **fortunate**.
Although children can easily learn to speak a second **language**/ with a native **accent**,/ adults are not as **fortunate**.
Although **children**/ can easily learn to speak a second language with a native **accent**,/ **adults**/ are not as **fortunate**.

There are many other possibilities. The word *fortunate* comes right before the period, and as the last content word, it receives focus in each version. There is also a connection between the pauses and other focus words since in all three versions, a focus word comes right before the comma. Nevertheless, it is important to keep in mind that due to emphasis, we cannot say that any particular word has to be the focus word even if it comes right before a period or a comma. Now consider some other versions of the same sentence:

> Although children can easily learn to speak a second language with a native accent, (disregard comma) adults are not as **fortunate**.
> Although children can easily learn **to**/ speak a **second**/ language with a native **accent**,/ adults are not **as**/ **fortunate**.

These version sound less natural. In the first version there is only one phrase, and although it is possible to produce the sentence this way, it is hard to imagine it sounding natural. In the second sentence, the phrase boundaries are in unnatural locations.

Speakers of English, therefore, have many options available to them, but some of them are probably much more likely to sound natural, and essentially come down to personal choice, while others might only work in extremely rare contexts, if at all.

Clients generally have good intuition about where a pause might not be natural, but there are several pointers that can help guide them. In general, there should not be a pause between articles, prepositions, and possessive pronouns and the nouns they precede, so it would not be typical to see a break between the words in the phrases *the car at home*, or *my friend*. In addition, infinitives are not normally separated, so there would not be a break in the middle of the infinitive *to do*. There is a little more variation when it comes to conjunctions, but phrases usually begin, rather than end with them, so "I wanted chips/ or pretzels," is more common than, "I wanted chips or/ pretzels." As in everything related to suprasegmentals, clients must use judgement since it is hard to find absolutes.

Clinicians can practice these concepts by having clients examine sets of sentences with different phrasal divisions to identify which ones sound natural, keeping in mind that it is hard to issue blanket statements that a particular version is impossible. Here are some example sentences to illustrate this type of task:

> Why don't you / ask / her about the party?
> Why don't you ask her / about the party?
> Why don't you / ask her about the party?

Clients can discuss which versions seem more likely to occur, and then the clinician can have them model the sentences to gets some good practice connecting other suprasegmental features such as intonation and linking. For example, the third sentence might be a good opportunity to practice emphasis by having the client put a high degree of stress on *you* to show an intended contrast. Appendix 9–3 features several other examples that clients can analyze.

This might also be a good place to discuss possible changes in meaning related to phrasing in conjunction with intonation. For example, clients can take phrases such as the two below and play around with various combinations that could produce entirely different meanings depending on where the pauses come, in conjunction with the overall prosody:

I called her honey
We sold twenty five dollar T-shirts

Note that punctuation is omitted to make it easier to visualize the possibilities. Although this is fun for clients and certainly something worth pointing out, it is less important overall than working on the connection of phrasing to naturalness.

Clients need to develop a good understanding of where they can break up the speech stream in order to sound more natural, and they also need to consider how long their phrases should be. There is a great deal of individual variation in how many words speakers include in a typical phrase, and the choice is highly dependent on context. Clinicians can work with clients to monitor the approximate number of words to produce between pauses in order to sound natural in various situations. There is an intelligibility connection here as well. Clients who are struggling to produce easily understood speech may benefit from producing shorter phrases, and this is especially true for those clients whose high rate of speech causes difficulties with intelligibility. There can be dramatic improvement when clients who sound like they are speaking too quickly use more phrases without significantly reducing their rate.

Clinicians should work with clients to develop an awareness of how phrasing connects to punctuation. Most accent training is designed to practice spontaneous speech, but clients may also need to read out loud, especially if they typically give presentations in their work. By taking a longer sentence and walking through several natural phrasing options, clinicians can probe clients' understanding of several important factors. For example, periods are basically automatic phrase boundary markers, so clients should watch for them carefully. Commas, on the other hand, are somewhat trickier since clients actually have a tendency to automatically pause when they see them, even when they are used by convention, as opposed to indicating a mandatory break. Clients should also understand that they have much more freedom to decide where they want to pause, and they can use the guidelines above related to naturalness as opposed to the punctuation on the page to make those decisions. Clinicians can point out that two native speakers reading the same exact text will typically use different phrasing.

When clients need to give their own presentations frequently, a good training technique is to have them mark out some of their planned pauses using slashes. This is also an excellent way to develop awareness for all clients, and it serves as a nice intermediate step in developing their awareness to monitor phrasing. This idea can be combined with some awareness building of where to place focus by having clients underline the word with tonic stress in each phrase.

# References

Dickerson, W. (2015). A NAIL in the coffin of stress-timed rhythm. In J. Levis, R. Mohamed, M. Qian, & Z. Zhou (Eds.), *Proceedings of the 6th Pronunciation in Second Language Learning and Teaching Conference* (pp. 183–193). Aimes, IA: Iowa State University.

Dickerson, W. (2016). A practitioner's guide to English rhythm: A return to confidence. In J. Levis, R. Mohamed, M. Qian, & Z. Zhou (Eds.), *Proceedings of the 7th Pronunciation in Second Language Learning and Teaching Conference* (pp. 39–50). Aimes, IA: Iowa State University.

Pike, K. (1945). *The intonation of American English.* Ann Arbor, MI: The University of Michigan Press.

Prator, C. (1972). *Manual of American English pronunciation.* New York, NY: Holt, Rinehart and Winston.

# Stress with Too/Either

Read each sentence in response to what you hear. Remember to stress the word that makes the most sense:

Example:

Sentence: He plays electric guitar too.

You hear: He plays acoustic guitar.

You say: He plays ELECTRIC guitar TOO.

1. He works with his sister too.
2. Ron works out at the gym on Tuesday too.
3. Karen studied in Budapest two years ago too.
4. My mother grew up in Chicago too.
5. It's expensive to buy property in California too.
6. She doesn't live near any Chinese restaurants either.
7. Walter didn't buy any shoes for his girlfriend either.
8. Ken wouldn't live in Colorado without his family either.
9. Sarah couldn't pass her chemistry class last semester either.
10. Dan has never taken his bike to work before either.

Prompts:

1. He works with his sister too.

   a. He works with his brother.

   b. He lives with his sister.

   c. She works with his sister.

   d. He works with John's brother.

2. Ron works out at the gym on Tuesday too.

    a. Ron works out at the gym on Monday.

    b. Ken works out at the gym on Tuesday.

    c. Ron works at the gym on Tuesday.

    d. Ron works at the hospital on Tuesday.

3. Karen studied in Budapest two years ago too.

    a. Karen studied in Prague two years ago.

    b. Karen worked in Budapest two years ago.

    c. Karen studied in Budapest last year.

    d. Roger studied in Budapest two years ago.

4. Ken's father had a house in Chicago too.

    a. Ken's mother had a house in Chicago.

    b. My father had a house in Chicago.

    c. Ken's father had a store in Chicago.

    d. Ken's father had a house in Boston.

5. It's expensive to buy property in California too.

    a. It's expensive to buy a business in California.

    b. It's expensive to buy property in New York.

    c. It's important to buy property in California.

    d. It's expensive to rent property in California.

6. She doesn't live near any Chinese restaurants either.

    a. He doesn't live near any Chinese restaurants.

    b. She doesn't work near any Chinese restaurants.

    c. She doesn't live near any Chinese stores.

    d. She doesn't live near any Japanese restaurants.

7. Walter didn't buy any shoes for his girlfriend either.

    a. Walter didn't buy any shoes for himself.

    b. Walter didn't buy any clothes for his girlfriend.

    c. Dave didn't buy any shoes for his girlfriend.

    d. Walter didn't buy any shoes for Don's girlfriend.

8. Ken wouldn't live in Colorado without his family either.

    a. Ken wouldn't live in Nevada without his family.

    b. Ken wouldn't work in Colorado without his family.

    c. Richard wouldn't work in Colorado without his family.

    d. Ken wouldn't live in Colorado with his family.

9.  Sarah couldn't pass her chemistry class last semester either.

    a. Sarah couldn't pass her chemistry class this semester.

    b. Sarah couldn't pass her math class last semester.

    c. Charlotte couldn't pass her chemistry class last semester.

    d. Sarah couldn't get an A in her chemistry class last semester.

10.  Dan has never taken his bike to work before either.

    a. Dan has never taken his bike from work before.

    b. Will has never taken his bike to work before.

    c. Dan has never taken his bike to the store before.

    d. Dan has never taken my bike to work before.

# 9–2

# Emphasis for Disagreement/ Agreement Worksheet

## A. Disagreement

Listen to the following sentences and then correct the information using contrastive stress. Remember that you can introduce your correction in a variety of ways, such as *No . . . ,* *Actually . . . , I always thought . . . , I'm sure that . . . ,* etcetera:

Example:  The sun rises in the west.

No, it actually rises in the EAST.

or

I think it SETS in the west.

1. Mt. Whitney is the tallest mountain in the world.
2. The Earth is the fourth planet from the sun.
3. The United States is the most populous country in the world.
4. A dime is worth 5 cents.
5. There are seven people in the room right now.
6. The Mississippi is the longest river in the world.
7. The Wright brothers invented the light bulb.
8. The chemical symbol for water is $CO_2$.
9. Peru and Bolivia are in Europe.
10. Smoking is good for your health.

## B. Agreement

Listen to the following sentences and agree with them. Remember to add auxiliaries when necessary:

Example:  I think Shakespeare wrote Hamlet.

You're right. He **did** write Hamlet.

1. I'm pretty sure Bucharest is the capital of Romania.
2. It's nice in here.
3. I think I have to buy a new car.
4. German is spoken in Austria.
5. They say that he's the one to talk to.
6. I feel like I'm overqualified for the job.
7. I guess you gave him a lot of money.
8. I think Mt. Everest is the tallest mountain in the world.
9. Mr. Smith has a lot of free time.
10. I think he used to live in Mali.

# 9–3

# Natural Phrasing

Decide which sentences have natural pauses. There may be more than one answer:

1.   If you / worked a little harder you might get / a raise.

   If you worked a little harder / you might / get a raise.

   If you worked / a little harder/ you might get a raise.

2.   Why don't you / ask / her about the party?

   Why don't you ask her / about the party?

   Why don't you / ask her about the party?

3.   Please let me / know before you go / home for the evening.

   Please / let me know / before you go home for the evening.

   Please let / me know / before you go home / for the evening.

4.   He bought a new laptop / on the weekend.

   He bought / a new laptop / on the weekend.

   He / bought a new laptop on the weekend.

5.   You're always / trying to / convince me / that I'm not a good writer.

   You're always trying / to convince me that / I'm not a good writer.

   You're always trying to convince me / that I'm not a / good writer.

# 10

# Connected Speech

## Overview of Connected Speech

When we speak, we constantly balance the need to be clear and natural. Most speech is spontaneous and connected, and this type of speech tends to shift more in the direction of sounding natural. Generally, it is understood that speech changes in more casual contexts, but native and non-native speakers alike tend to downplay the amount of change that occurs in even relatively formal situations. The truth is that as soon as English sounds come into contact with one another, they affect each other, and the results can be profound. While the terms *informal, casual, spontaneous* and many others are useful in describing connected speech, perhaps it is best to simply call it *natural speech* to emphasize how pervasive it is and how important it is to master.

Native speakers are aware of some, but not most, features of connected speech. Our writing system uses contractions to highlight some of the more obvious changes that occur, but in most cases the written word does not reflect what happens in the speech stream. In some cases, we use eye dialect forms such as *gonna* and *didja*, but these are generally used to indicate excessive casualness or slang. In reality, reduced forms are all around us, from everyday encounters to board rooms and conference calls. Clients will benefit not only from having an awareness of the features of connected speech, but they are also likely to find that applying them helps them become more effective communicators in virtually every context.

## Linking Consonants

Spoken English sounds much more like the music of a violin than a piano, and this may be somewhat different from languages spoken by our clients. There is a connecting effect that occurs in the sounds of a word to produce allophonic variations, and sometimes the effect is strong enough to approach the realm of the phoneme. As words are joined within a phrase, the phonemes within them tend to become linked, and although this process is noticeable, native speakers are generally not conscious of it. Non-native speakers, especially those whose L1 does not undergo the same process, benefit from awareness building and practice at the word and phrase level. We can define *linking* as the connection of sounds across word boundaries, but at times we will also look within words, because analogous processes occur between and within words. Linking can be divided into three types: CV, CC, and VV. CV linking describes situations in which one word ends in a consonant and the next word starts with a vowel, or vice versa. We can also add situations in which a word ends in two consonants and the next word starts with a vowel, since this allows a split of the consonants into separate syllables, so that in a phrase such as "fix it," the words can become resyllabified as /fɪk.sɪt/. CC is used to describe liaison between two consonants and VV between two vowels. CC linking is the most complex since there are so many possible combinations and patterns, and clients can work on this phenomenon in stages. Clients often ask when linking occurs, and the best short answer is probably whenever possible, but it is important to point out that when it occurs, it occurs within a phrase, so this feature fits in well with work on thought groups and phrasing.

Sanskrit gives us the word *sandhi* to refer to changes that occur at word boundaries, and the early phonetician Panini analyzed its role in that language over 2,000 years ago (Hyman, 2009). Nevertheless, formal research on linking and second language acquisition began relatively late when compared to other aspects of suprasegmental phonology involved in L2 acquisition. Hieke (1984) was one of the first to examine linking in detail, and he found that out of every 100 syllables produced in casual speech, there are about 12 CV links in which the consonant connected two vowels across word boundaries. The fact that only one type of linking was considered and found to be so prominent is evidence that this is a significant feature of connected speech. Moreover, his research showed that while native English speakers turned 80% of potential links of this type into actual links, native speakers of German acquiring English did so only 54% of the time. When we consider that some languages allow only minimal linking, the importance of linking in English becomes all the more obvious. A study by Alameen (2007) looked at consonant-vowel and vowel-vowel linking in native versus non-native speakers and found similar results. In addition, that study did not find a difference in the low rates of linking for beginning, compared to intermediate non-native speakers. In short, linking is an extremely common process in English that is vital for natural sounding English speech.

## CV Linking

When English vowels and consonants come together in a phrase they link up so naturally that it might be difficult to know where one word begins and another ends if we did not have prior knowledge of word boundaries. Compare the single word *banana* /bənænə/ to an article plus noun such as *an apple* [ənæpl̩]. If we said these words to someone who was unfamiliar with English, they would really have no way of knowing that *banana* was said without an article and *an apple* was said with an article. In other languages, it might be more obvious where word boundaries occur because these languages use less linking. The links are so strong in English that they have even led to changes in our words. You might be surprised to learn that when we say *an apron* we are using a new form of the older version of the word which was *a napron*. Over time, listeners forgot that "napron" starts with an "n" because of this linking effect!

### Linking with /n/

Perhaps the easiest starting point for developing clients' awareness of linking effects is to focus on words in which a single consonant separates two vowels, as in *an apple*. Clients generally have little difficulty producing a word such as *banana* with a continuous airstream, but there is an interference effect when they see two words and create an artificial separation between them. Many clients say a short phrase like *in an hour* with distinct pauses between the words, and they may even add or substitute a glottal stop between words. This is especially problematic for tonal language speakers. A good exercise to develop awareness and provide practice opportunities is to have clients produce phrases with the indefinite article *an* plus a word beginning in a vowel, such as this:

> Say each phrase without pausing between the words:
> an orange
> an equation
> an hourglass
> an obstacle
> an igloo

This is a relatively straightforward exercise that rarely poses a challenge for students once they are given guidance. After succeeding with these prompts, clients can be given words that begin with vowels and asked to add the article themselves to promote generalization. The /n/ is usually a good place to start with clients who have more serious difficulties connecting words, and a logical extension is to move from the article plus noun to two- and three-word combinations that feature the same effect without the article (e.g., *in an elevator, on an even angle*).

### Linking with /t/

Another important topic to address is the allophonic variation in phrases where /t/ becomes intervocalic and is produced as an alveolar tap. It only makes sense to address this subject after the client is familiar with the rules for the tap and how to produce it. Clients need to know that this between-words effect is not fixed, and there is considerably more variation in comparison to intervocalic /t/ within a word. While the word *water* will virtually always feature a tap, a phrase such as *hit it out* may be produced with a /t/ between *hit* and *it,* and between *it* and *out* in very careful speech or if the speaker chooses to pause between the words for effect. Although producing a strong /t/ and not a tap in these contexts may be rare, it is more common between words than within them. Clinicians can model different versions of sentences to give clients a feel for the possibilities. For example, in the sentence, "I owed a lot of money to Tim," the clinician can model a version where there is a tap between *money* and *to* and another version where there is a /t/.

To practice linking with the tap, clients can be given short phrases and asked to connect and produce the words without pausing, such as the examples below:

> Say the following phrases with a connecting tap:
> eat at eight
> what it is
> got out at eleven

Separable phrasal verbs (such as *pick up*, *knock off*) are especially useful to practice because when they are used with the pronoun *it*, the resulting intervocalic context will produce a natural tap in American English. These also represent good opportunities to work on generalization as shown in this sample activity:

> Listen to a statement, and then ask a question starting with *when* and using the pronoun *it*:
> Example: I hit the ball out of the park.
> Response: "When did you hit it out of the park?"
> Prompts:
> I put the answer on the board.
> I set up the equipment.
> She shut down the machine.

### Intervocalic Linking with Other Consonants

The same techniques from above can be applied to work with other consonants; clients should have exposure to a wide range of combinations to determine which ones are problematic. They can practice with phrases such as *judge it*, *pick up*, and *for every*. Clinicians can practice linking with phonemes that a particular client may have trouble with in other contexts, so a Japanese client can work on linking with /ɹ/, and a Spanish speaker can focus on /z/. With voiced sounds, linking provides an optimal context to practice production, so working with Spanish-speaking clients on their /z/ during linking activities might provide a facilitative context.

When working on linking, a resyllabification technique can be useful, especially when working with clients whose L1 is a tonal language. If clients are not producing the final consonant in a word, as in /faɪ/ for *five*, they can use linking to bridge the gap. Often clients with these phonotactic difficulties drop the final sound in a word produced in isolation, but by shifting the position of the phoneme, they have a better chance of producing the phrase accurately. For example, they can practice producing a phrase such as *five oh* after being instructed to focus on producing it as a combination of /faɪ/ and /voʊ/ as opposed to /faɪv/ and /oʊ/. By resyllabifying in this way, clients produce more accurate linking and will possibly be able to extend these gains to produce the final consonant at a later point when encountering it in a different context. Telling time is another good way to create practice opportunities. Clients can view prompts as shown below. For example, 5:09 should be produced as /faɪvoʊnaɪn/:

Read the time out loud using oh for zero:
5:09
6:03
4:07
8:02

As an extension of the idea of resyllabification, clients can work on linking phrases in which the first word ends in a two-element cluster, and the second word begins with a vowel. For example, in the case of the phrase *find it*, ask them to focus on producing it as /faɪn/ plus /dɪt/. If clients pause excessively between the words, gradually prompt them to connect them. Try combining work on producing difficult clusters with practice on linking. Here are some examples of possible prompts:

> Link the following word pairs by splitting the consonants:
> Example: *send it* = "sen" "dit" Try not to pause between the words.
> ask it
> fix everything
> fork over
> washed again
> left out

Appendix 10–1 provides activities related to CV linking.

## CC Linking

Consonant to consonant linking can be the most challenging for clients because so much variation occurs when different types of sounds connect. In addition, several different types of processes occur, such as elision and assimilation, so CC linking is best tackled in stages. Rather than including assimilation and elision in work on linking, they can be addressed as separate topics.

### *Extending Consonants*

In some cases, when consonants connect, especially in the case of adjacent fricatives, the sounds are simply extended. In the phrase *kiss someone*, there would generally not be a break between the two words, and the /s/ would be extended. It is often easiest to begin with pairs like this, where the phonemes are identical, and then extend the idea to pairs which differ in voicing. Note that there may be some assimilation effect if there is a voicing difference between the fricatives. Here are some examples of prompts:

> miss something (identical phonemes)
> quiz someone (voicing difference in phonemes)
> loose zipper (voicing difference in phonemes)

Determine how naturally clients produce these links; there may be different types of assimilation taking place. For example, the /z/ in *quiz* may be partially or completely devoiced before the /s/ in *someone*. When fricatives produced in different places align, the transition is not as easy, but speakers generally produce them without an abrupt break, and the most important concept for clients to master is the uninterrupted connection between the sounds. Clients can practice with pairs such as those that follow:

wish farewell
slash that
five thousand

### Hold and Release

When two consonants line up and the first one is a stop, native speakers generally hold the stop and produce the next consonant. For example, in the phrase *stop panicking*, speakers tend to hold the /p/ in *stop* and then release the /p/ at the beginning of *panicking*. Similarly, in the phrase *keep talking* speakers hold the /p/ and release the /t/. This effect occurs when other types of consonants follow the stop too, and clients can practice any number of combinations to develop awareness of the connections that occur between words. Example practice phrases might include:

quit firing
lip service
black zipper

Other changes may occur due to assimilatory processes or other coarticulation effects, and clinicians should highlight anything of interest as clients produce these combinations. For example, the combination in *what should* produces the affricate /tʃ/, while the phrase *could we* could result in the /d/ being released since the following sound is an approximant, and *was she* could result in assimilation of the /s/ to the /ʃ/.

## The Glottal Stop

Instead of holding a final /t/ when it abuts a consonant in the word that follows it, native speakers might substitute a glottal stop. This usually occurs if the next word starts with a stop. For example, the phrase *cute baby* could be produced as [kjuʔbeɪbi]. Although clients may be hesitant to use a glottal stop themselves, they should practice it to build awareness and provide options. Sample prompts could be:

hot dog
bat boy
fit tight

This effect can also occur with /d/ before voiced stops, as in *good girl*. Appendix 10–2 provides a series of prompts to practice these connections.

## Assimilation

When two or more consonants come into contact, the changes tend to be more complicated. One process that often occurs is assimilation, in which one or more sounds change to become more similar. When we looked at English -*s* and -*ed* endings, the assimilation was progressive because the final sound of the word affected the voicing of the ending, but in connected speech the process generally happens in reverse, and is called regressive assimilation. In some cases, the effect may be barely noticeable, but you can point it out to clients so that they are aware of an easier, more natural way to produce certain combinations. For example, when we say, "I can buy some," the /n/ in *can* will probably be produced as /m/ since the next sound is a /b/, which is also bilabial. If we say, "I can go," the /n/ in *can* will probably become /ŋ/ because the sound /g/ in *go* is velar. Another type of example is when /z/ comes before /ʃ/ as when *was she* becomes /wʌʒʃi/. In these cases, the place of articulation changed, but voicing can be affected as well. In the phrase *have to* the /v/ in *have* is almost always /f/ because the following /t/ is unvoiced. In some cases, the sound essentially assimilates until it disappears, as in *lemme* for *let me*. As sounds connect during practice activities, keep an eye out for any possible assimilations to help clients develop their awareness of them.

At other times, the assimilations are more noticeable, and both native speakers and clients are conscious of them. For example, in a phrase such as *what's your name*, the /s/ + /j/ often coalesce into the /tʃ/ affricate, and it sounds something like [wʌtʃɚneɪm]. Both clinicians and clients tend to be averse to working on this aspect of spontaneous speech, but it is clearly important for clients to note. As with all aspects of accent work, clients benefit from understanding the features of natural speech, and as they monitor the speech stream around them, they can identify which features might help their communication and in which contexts. Clients report that they gain an appreciation of the frequency of these forms even as part of what might be considered deliberate, or formal, speech.

Palatalization occurs when alveolar fricatives precede the /j/ and are moved further back to the postalveolar position. This assimilatory process is very common since the high frequency pronouns *you* and *your* both start with /j/. Table 10–1 illustrates how this process works. Because the *s* ending is so common in English, it helps to look at what happens when words end in either /ts/ or /dz/ precede a /j/, as shown in Table 10–2.

**Table 10–1.** Assimilation

| Phoneme | + /j/ = | Example |
|---------|---------|---------|
| /s/ | /ʃ/ | bless you /blɛʃu/ |
| /t/ | /tʃ/ | bet you /bɛtʃu/ or /bɛtʃə/ |
| /z/ | /ʒ/ | was your /wʌʒɚ/ |
| /d/ | /dʒ/ | would you /wʊdʒu/ or /wʊdʒə/ |

**Table 10–2.** /ts/ and /dz/ + /j/ Assimlation

| Phonemes | + /j/ = | Example |
|----------|---------|---------|
| /ts/ | /tʃ/ | he hates you [hiheɪtʃu] |
| /dz/ | /dʒ/ | she needs you [ʃinidʒu] |

Many English modals and auxiliaries end with /d/ (e.g., *would, should, did*), so this is often a logical place to practice some typical assimilations that occur with these words. Clients can practice saying the full forms to represent the way they might sound in deliberate speech, and then work on producing more natural versions. Table 10–3 shows some possibilities for auxiliaries and modals.

## Pronoun Reduction

Another typical feature of connected speech occurs when native speakers drop the initial /h/ (and sometimes /ð/ as well) of words. This occurs most commonly with pronouns, but it also happens in other words in less deliberate speech. Clients should be aware of this process because of its connection to linking, and because it affects the naturalness of their speech if they overpronounce the /h/ in their pronouns. For example, a client might analyze a phrase such as *did he* as being a combination of two consonants, but in reality, native speakers treat it as a CV link because the /h/ is dropped, as shown in Table 10–4.

**Table 10–3.** Auxiliary Assimilations

| Auxiliary | Clear | Natural | Example Sentence | Pronunciation |
|-----------|-------|---------|------------------|---------------|
| Do you | [duju] | [ʤə] | Do you see me? | [ʤəsimi] |
| Don't you | [doʊntju] | [dɔnʧə] | Don't you know? | [dɔnʧənoʊ] |
| Did you | [dɪdju] | [dɪʤə] | Did you do it? | [dɪʤəduʷɪt] |
| Didn't you | [dɪdn̩tju] | [dɪdn̩ʧə] | Didn't you go? | [dɪdn̩ʧəgoʊ] |

**Table 10–4.** Dropped /h/ in Pronouns

| Pronoun | Clear | Natural | Example Sentence | Pronunciation |
|---------|-------|---------|------------------|---------------|
| he | [hi] | [i] | What did he want? | What did "e" want? [wəɾɾiwant̚] |
| him | [hɪm] | [əm] | I told him. | I told "im". [aɪtɔldəm] |
| her | [hɝ] | [ɚ] | He likes her. | He likes "er". [hilaɪksɚ] |
| them | [ðɛm] | [əm] | She likes them. | She likes "em" [ʃilaɪksəm] |

Note that the only subject pronoun in the table is *he* and that is reduced unless it is at the beginning of a phrase, so we would never delete the *h* in a sentence like "He is eating lunch," but we would delete it in a sentence like "Why is (h)e eating lunch?" if the preceding word is part of the same phrase. Also notice that the reduced forms for *him* and *them* are basically the same, so we use context to determine the meaning. Appendix 10–3 offers several sentences that feature assimilation, and clinicians should help clients develop awareness of the assimilation when producing spontaneous speech and reading passages.

## The Rule of Three and Endings

### Elision

When three or more consonants connect intervocalically or postvocalically, the middle consonant often disappears, especially when it is an unvoiced stop. Native speakers use this process to keep the speech stream fluent, but non-native speakers often avoid it and sound choppy. For example, when a native speaker produces the phrase *fast car*, three consonants align /stk/ and the /t/ is usually elided, resulting in [fæskaɚ]. Non-native speakers, on the other hand, might produce this as two distinct words with a released /t/ at the end of *fast*. Although this would be intelligible to listeners, it won't sound natural, and listeners will focus on how the message is conveyed as opposed to the message itself. Clients can practice dropping these medial consonants in phrases such as the following:

most common /stk/ → /sk/
text message /kstm/ → /ksm/
prompt delivery /mptd/ → /mpd/ (Note that the /p/ can also be omitted but the vowel will be shortened. Compare natural versions of *prom delivery* and *prompt delivery*.)

When these combinations occur, there is no hard and fast rule about which sounds are elided, and native speakers always have the option of producing all of the sounds in careful speech. Table 10–5 illustrates some examples in both citation form and more natural speech.

This feature can be practiced with linking in connected speech and in individual words, especially words with "s" endings. Clients may need encouragement to practice the more natural versions of these words, as they have been trained to overpronounce endings to enhance intelligibility. The goal is always to achieve a balance, but clinicians should push clients to practice forms that require time to incorporate into clients' active speech to help them develop awareness and to give them more range. Appendix 10–4 provides practice with this type of elision.

It is perhaps more important to ensure that clients understand that although overpronouncing the endings can make them sound less natural, dropping the final *s* because of difficulty with final clusters is a mistake that will be noticed immediately and probably considered as a grammatical error, which may be rated more harshly than overpronouncing. To illustrate differences between native and non-native speech, clinicians can demonstrate two typical ways of producing the word *tests* in a sentence such as, "I took three tests last week.":

Non-native: [tɛst]
Native: [tɛsː]

In both cases a consonant was dropped, but in the non-native version, the ending is missing. Always advise clients of the importance of producing endings in English, especially the *s*. One exception to this rule of three involves the interdental fricatives, as these will often disappear when followed by an /s/, as shown in Table 10–6. Once again, it is important to produce these words naturally, so if a client is speaking too slowly or having any difficulties with the other segmentals in these words, it may be too early to encourage this process.

**Table 10–5.** Citation Form Versus Natural Speech

| Process | Example Word or Phrase phras | Citation Form pronunciation | Natural Speech pronunciation |
|---|---|---|---|
| ndz → nz | sands | [sændz] | [sænz] |
| | round zone | [ɹaʊndzoʊn] | [ɹaʊnzoʊn] |
| nθs→ts | months | [mʌnθs] | [mʌnts] |
| | a month somewhere | [əmʌnθsʌmwɛɚ] | [əmʌntsəmwɛɚ] |
| sts→sː | tests | [tɛsts] | [tɛsː] |
| | best seat | [bɛstsit] | [bɛsːit] |
| sks→ sː | asks | [æsks] | [æsː] |
| | ask something | [æsksʌmpθɪŋ] | [æsːʌnθɪŋ] |
| pts→psː | accepts | [ɛksɛpts] | [ɛksɛps] |
| | intercept something | [ɪntɚsɛptsʌmpθɪŋ] | [ɪɾɚsɛpsʌnθɪŋ] |
| fts→fsː | shifts | [ʃɪfts] | [ʃɪfs] |
| | lifts him | [lɪftshɪm] | [lɪfsɪm] |

**Table 10–6.** "th" Elision

| ðz→z | clothes | kloʊðz | kloʊz |
|---|---|---|---|
| θs→s | paths | pæθs | pæs |

### Linking of the Regular Past

Consonant elision helps clients produce the regular past tense in connected speech more naturally. For infinitives ending in /t,d/, the extra syllable added when producing the past tense sets it apart from its present tense counterpart, and when native speakers use other regular past forms before a word that begins with a vowel, it is easy to distinguish it from the present tense. "I watched a show," sounds very different from, "I watch a show," because there is a consonant sequence of /ʧt/ between the words *watched* and *show* in the past tense, but in the present, there is only the single consonant /ʧ/. On the other hand, if the next word starts with a consonant, then there is normally elision, so because, "I watched the show," now features three consecutive consonants /ʧtð/, the /t/ often elides. Thus, there is often no difference between, "I watch the show" and "I watched the show," in normal natural speech. Native speakers typically believe they are producing all of the consonants in this context, and that is always an option in deliberate speech, but the reality is that they rarely do. Non-native speakers tend to overpronounce, and to carefully produce grammatical endings, but because this sequence is difficult, they are likely to pause between words, so when they say, "I watched the show," there is often a break between *watched* and *show* that is rare for native speakers to produce. Appendix 10–5 offers prompts to draw attention to this type of elision in connected speech. The key to sounding natural is for non-native speakers (if they are speaking at a normal rate) to produce the regular past tense in the same way as the present tense if the following word begins with a consonant, just as native speakers do.

# Linking Vowels

An often-overlooked feature of English is the linking that takes place when two vowels connect either within a word or across word boundaries. To illustrate, in the word *pronunciation*, there is no break between the vowels represented by the letters *i* and *a*, and instead a glide allows the voicing to continue. In narrow transcription a superscript /j/ can be inserted to show this allophonic variation [pɹənəntsiʲeɪʃn̩]. Speakers of other languages might stop the airflow between the two vowels, which sounds unnatural to our ears. This same effect occurs in connected speech when we say something like, "I can't see anyone," where there is a /j/ glide between *see* and *anyone*. The /j/ glide is inserted after front vowels, and the /w/ is inserted after back vowels. In the sentence, "I need to do it," *do it* can be transcribed as [duʷɪt]. If clients stop the airflow between these two words, their speech sounds choppy. There is, however, no link for the back vowel /ɑ/, and you can hear how unnatural it sounds to insert a /j/ or /w/ between *saw* and *it* in the sentence, "I saw it." In this case, a glottal stop serves as a transition between the vowels. So ingrained is this effect that native speakers are rarely aware of it on any level. If you ask a native speaker to compare *you ate* and *you wait* in normal connected speech, you are likely to cause some reflection.

The linking effect that occurs with the definite article *the* is a nice way to practice this concept since many non-native speakers may already be connecting it with a /j/

glide. When native speakers add *the* to a word, they normally produce it with a schwa in connected speech if the following word starts with a consonant, but if it starts with a vowel, they have two choices. Some speakers produce *the* with the /i/ vowel and then link it up to the next word with the glide, as in *the end* [ðiʲɛnd]. Other speakers, depending on dialect or idiolect, simply keep the schwa and connect the vowels without a linking glide or with a light glottal stop, as in [ðəʔɛnd]. Clinicians can practice this process by asking clients to place a definite article before a prompt word and link it with /j/. Make sure they know that there is quite a bit of variation in native speech, and that they can use the glottal stop version if they prefer. Since this is such a common process, encourage them to focus on each listener they encounter to determine which version the speaker normally uses, which will heighten awareness of linking.

Another good practice technique is to have the client spell words. First, it might be good to review the names of the consonants quickly to point out how English letter names tend to go back and forth between starting with the sound and ending with a vowel as in *t* /ti/ and starting with a vowel and ending with the sound as in *s* /ɛs/. Because of this, when we spell words, vowels often align and in normal speech they are linked with a /j/ glide. On a side note, I sometimes point out how strange our name for the letter *h* /eɪtʃ/ is since in American English it does not normally contain the actual sound the letter normally makes, namely the /h/. If we spell out *peas* for example, we would have something like [piʲiʲeɪʲɛs]. Clients should know that in the real world, it is probably best to slow down and spell things out unnaturally to avoid any confusion that relates to lower intelligibility or the unfamiliarity of listeners with the word being spelled (since in many cases it will be the client's name). Spelling is a fun awareness-builder that provides some good practice with linking.

A nice extension of this activity is to move to another typical combination of vowels, when the pronouns *he, she, they, I* precede a verb that begins with a vowel since this is also a common occurrence. Examples to practice are phrases like *I ate* or *he earns*. Clinicians can then contrast these forms with the same verbs plus *you*. *You* has a back vowel, so it links with /w/, and not the /j/. Provide a verb and a pronoun as prompts, and have clients connect them with a glide. For example, if the prompts are *earn* and *he*, the client says *he earns* using a /j/ glide between the words, but if the prompts are *earn* and *you*, the words are linked with a /w/. The same verbs can be used with both types of pronouns to make the contrast more obvious. Appendix 10–6 offers examples of several different vowel linking exercise.

## Putting It All Together

Connected speech processes can be addressed at any stage of training since they are such a pervasive element of natural communication. Many SLPs may feel that some of these processes should come only after clients have established good intelligibility, but there is a good case to be made for initiating the conversation on this topic at an early stage. Clients have probably heard many of these forms but are unsure about why natives use them, so building awareness gives them more control. As they listen to the speech around them, clients are bound to hear these patterns often, and by bringing them to the foreground, clinicians help them develop more natural speech.

# References

Alameen, G. (2007). *The use of linking by native and non-native speakers of American English* (Unpublished master's thesis). Aimes, IA: Iowa State University.

Hieke, A. E. (1984). Linking as a marker of fluent speech. *Language and Speech. 27*, 343–354

Hyman, M.D. (2009). From Pāṇinian sandhi to finite state calculus. In: Huet G., Kulkarni A., Scharf P. (eds) *Sanskrit computational linguistics. ISCLS 2007, ISCLS 2008. Lecture notes in computer science*, (vol. 5402). Springer, Berlin, Heidelberg

# 10-1

# CV Linking

**Linking Consonants and Vowels**

Put *a* or *an* in front of each word and make sure that you link them up without pausing:

| | |
|---|---|
| rose | aviator |
| operator | zipper |
| alligator | riverboat |
| lollipop | laser |
| rhinoceros | overachiever |

**Telling Time**

Read out the time and link your sounds. Example 5:06 = five_o_six [faɪvoʊsɪks]:

| | |
|---|---|
| 6:04 | 5:05 |
| 7:09 | 9:02 |
| 4:07 | 12:04 |
| 11:06 | 1:07 |
| 1:03 | 10:05 |

**Linking with /n/**

1. It was a one in a million opportunity.
2. "An apple a day" is an idiom in English.
3. In an annual report, there is an entry for an investment.
4. In any nation, there is an issue in everyone's focus.
5. I won an event in an aerobics contest.
6. You know, in an hour I can answer.

7.  If there was a need to know I noted it in a report.
8.  Anne and Alex phone in at 8 every evening.
9.  My zone is 109091.
10. An actor and an agent are in on the deal.

## Linking with /r/

1.  Calls for Rory or Esther are routed through there.
2.  He read her a really long story for an hour.
3.  They are in the register under a different name.
4.  I need a car and a radio right away.
5.  I hear everything there is to hear before I react.

## Linking with /t/
Circle the possible flaps in the following sentences and then practice saying them:

1.  I sat around the house at eight o'clock.
2.  I ate at Otto's and did it again at eleven.
3.  I owed a lot of money to Tim.
4.  I ought to take it out of here.
5.  Tell Matt about it at our meeting.
6.  He hit it at an angle.
7.  I taught it at a workshop without a problem.
8.  She put out a call to let it in.
9.  We put in some time to set up the stage, but it isn't what it ought to be.
10. If we eat at eleven, we'll sit at a table.

# 10-2

# Sample Consonant Linking Worksheet

## Splitting Consonants

First mark a slash between the two consonants you can split. Then practice saying the words:

| | |
|---|---|
| hand over | fork over |
| work it out | bulk order |
| drink up | slipped on |
| passed out | talked it through |
| help out | storm in |

## Extending Consonants

| | |
|---|---|
| fourth Thursday | come Monday |
| clear reason | call letters |
| tough final | above Venice |
| was zipping | wash shirts |
| toss something | has zippers |

## Hold and Release

| | |
|---|---|
| keep taking | chip through |
| skip town | flip down |
| back together | bad back |
| had time | Cape Town |
| put down | rub through |

## Glottal Stops

| | |
|---|---|
| cute baby | catnap |
| fat guy | potluck |
| batboy | cut class |

# 10-3

# Assimilation

Practice with the following phrases:

Was she there?

What did you do?

What's your number?

It's your party.

Pass your tests.

It hits your head.

Let me do it.

I bet you're tired.

What's your name?

Where's your sister?

Give me another piece.

I want you to know.

Would you like one?

Do you really like him?

I did your homework.

She was his friend.

# 10-4

# The Rule of Three

**Rule of Three Practice**

Reduce the final clusters in the following words by applying the rule of three:

1. desks
2. facts
3. asks
4. corrupts
5. months

6. mouths
7. crafts
8. scientists
9. adapts
10. lists

**Practice Sentences**

Try to reduce the highlighted clusters. Make sure to pronounce final *s*!

1. La<u>st</u> <u>Ch</u>ri<u>stm</u>a<u>s</u> I went to Co<u>stc</u>o and a<u>sked</u> for a tool that sa<u>nds</u> de<u>sks</u>.
2. If he atte<u>mpts</u> the ta<u>sks</u>, he acce<u>pts</u> the ri<u>sks</u>.
3. She insi<u>sts</u> that their stre<u>ngths</u> are the de<u>pths</u> of their characters.
4. Two fi<u>fths</u> times six twe<u>lfths</u> is twelve sixtie<u>ths</u>.
5. If he a<u>sks</u> you about the te<u>sts</u> make sure she assi<u>sts</u> you in your respon<u>se</u>.
6. If he spe<u>nds</u> six mo<u>nths</u> collecting fa<u>cts</u>, he'll go to great le<u>ngths</u> to deny it.
7. She be<u>nds</u> and dri<u>fts</u> with the wi<u>nds</u> while he re<u>sts</u>.
8. They left their clo<u>thes</u> in piles along the pa<u>ths</u> to their houses.

# 10-5

# Linking the Regular Past

Practice saying the two sentences so that there is a clear difference between them:

| Present | Past |
|---|---|
| We need a new car. | We needed a new car. |
| I live in Wisconsin. | I lived in Wisconsin. |
| They reside in New Jersey. | They resided in New Jersey. |
| We play every year. | We played every year. |
| I know that you love it. | I know that you loved it. |
| I laugh out loud. | I laughed out loud. |
| We decide on Thursday. | We decided on Thursday. |
| You watch a lot of TV. | You watched a lot of TV. |

Practice saying these phrases naturally so that they sound exactly alike. Don't pause after the past tense ending:

| Present | Past |
|---|---|
| They love to play soccer. | They loved to play soccer. |
| I replace the tire. | I replaced the tire. |
| I buzz the buzzer. | I buzzed the buzzer. |
| You watch the news. | You watched the news. |
| We plug the leak. | We plugged the leak. |

APPENDIX

# 10-6

# Vowel Linking Exercises

**The + Vowel**
Put the word *the* before each word and pronounce it as [ði]. Remember to link with /j/:

1. artist
2. elevator
3. engineer
4. office
5. internet

6. aggravation
7. unimportance
8. air conditioner
9. isolation
10. action

**You and I**
Place *you* and then *I* in front of each verb and make sure to link with /j/ or /w/:

1. act
2. organize
3. ate
4. attempt
5. oil

6. invent
7. eat
8. ooze
9. outlast
10. own

**Insert /j/ or /w/ in the appropriate place**
Example: g o ʷi n g    r e ʲa l i z e

| | | |
|---|---|---|
| weighing | see it | you ate |
| doing | go onto | I owe one |
| she is | pronunciation | tie it |
| biology | triangle | through art |
| reactivate | two each | no answer |

## Linking and Spelling

p – e – n

d – u – e – l

b – o – i – l

q – u – e – e – n

t – o – e – s

c – o – i – n

# 11

# Getting Started

Accent modification is truly one of the hidden treasures of our profession. It provides a wonderful avenue for SLPs to apply the insights, experience, and training they have in working with communicative disorders to an amazing group of clients with communication differences. It is especially rewarding to help clients make changes that can allow them to be as successful when speaking in their new language as they are in their mother tongue. Although much of this chapter focuses on getting a start in accent modification, details about running a business or opening a private practice are outside the scope of this book. Fortunately, there are many resources available on entrepreneurship and marketing, and this chapter focuses on the initial steps for SLPs planning to enter the field as well as some ideas for graduate students who will be working in university clinics before they begin their careers.

## Getting More Training

SLPs are well-trained, highly motivated, and driven to find the answers they need to improve their skills. While the aim of this book is to provide a good first step into the world of accent modification, SLPs are advised to find additional resources to maximize their capabilities. The first step should always be a solid familiarity with the basics of English phonology, and SLPs will often benefit most from dusting off their phonetics textbook and reviewing the material. There are also countless other avenues to get more training. Some are offered as part of a particular program, and a handful of these are described below, and there are also webinars and courses offered for continuing education units (CEUs) available through ASHA and other organizations. Because these courses come and go, it is easiest to simply research them through the ASHA website (http://www.asha.org) or an internet search. Companies that provide online CEUs for SLPs generally have introductory and intermediate courses focusing on accent modification. The annual ASHA convention often features talks on accent modification and offer an excellent opportunity to network with other professionals in the field. In addition, the yearly ASHA Connect conference provides additional opportunities to network and develop skills. Your state association for SLPs may also offer talks on accent modification and additional opportunities to connect.

ASHA's website features a wealth of information about every aspect of our field, and accent modification is no exception. ASHA continues to develop and expand its website and two sections of particular interest to most readers of this book are the Accent Modification Practice Portal at https://www.asha.org/Practice-Portal/Professional-Issues/Accent-Modification/ and the Private Practice in Speech-Language Pathology page at https://www.asha.org/slp/ppresources/. The Accent Modification Practice Portal includes a discussion of key issues and some helpful resources, and the Private Practice page discusses topics such as practice management, reimbursement, and ethical considerations. The Multicultural Affairs and Resources page https://www.asha.org/practice/multicultural/ has many useful links, such as the Phonemic Inventories and Linguistic Information Across Languages page at https://www.asha.org/practice/multicultural/Phono/ and the Speech Accent Archive at http://accent.gmu.edu/browse_native.php, which was discussed in Chapter 3 on assessment. This archive is an impressive collection of native and non-native English speech samples that clinicians can use to investigate accents and dialects. One final note concerning ASHA resources, Special Interest Group 14 on Cultural and Linguistic Diversity is worth joining for those involved in accent modification, especially for access to the Perspectives journal and its online community, which is a discussion forum where accent and dialect questions, as well as many other issues related to cultural and linguistic diversity are addressed.

Before providing more information on resources available to SLPs, it is important to point out the benefits of getting additional training in TESOL. SLPs pride themselves on their communication and language skills, and it often takes some humility to recognize that exceptional skills in one's L1 have only a limited connection to the ability to explain to adult second language learners the rules and patterns of a mother tongue acquired subconsciously from infancy. Native speakers who pride themselves on their grammar skills are generally referring to usage issues related to style and not to an awareness of the intricacies of their language, which typically confound non-native speakers. To illustrate, consider how you might explain the following aspects of English to a second language learner:

- We can say, "I like to read historical fiction," or "I like reading historical fiction," without changing the meaning, but we say, "I decided to go to the beach," and not "I decided going to the beach," and we say, "I enjoy skiing," but not "I enjoy to ski." How would you explain this to a non-native speaker? How would you explain the difference in meaning between, "I remembered buying her a present," and "I remembered to buy her a present"? Can you name other verbs that function this way?

- We can say, "I picked up my children from school," or "I picked my children up from school," but we can only say, "I picked them up from school," and not "I picked up them from school." We can say, "I ran into my friend at the mall," and "I ran into her at the mall," but we can't say, "I ran my friend into at the mall," or "I ran her into at the mall." What term is used to describe a verb plus preposition such as *pick up* or *run into* and how would you explain their various usage patterns to a language learner?

- A client reports to you that she heard the following sentences during the week: "I really like red wine," "I'd like a red wine," and "I didn't like the red wine." Her language does not use articles, so she wants you to explain the use of the indefinite article, the definite article, and no article in the three sentences. She also wants you to explain when to use articles with place names. Why do we say, *the Czech republic*, and *the Philippines*, but not *the China*? Why is it *the Nile* or *the Nile river*, but then we say, *Lake Erie*, not *the Erie*, *the lake Erie*, or *the Erie lake*?

Native speakers do not have to give much (if any) thought to these issues because of the way we absorb the fundamental grammar of our language, but they exemplify the types of questions that may arise when working with non-native speakers. Many SLPs focus purely on phonology and prefer clients who do not present with significant difficulties in other aspects of second language acquisition, such as syntax or semantics. Other SLPs treat grammar and vocabulary as equals in bridging the gap in clients' English proficiency. For SLPs planning to address all aspects of English, additional training is essential. While SLPs who are native speakers can always provide models and use their grammaticality judgment when helping clients master English syntax, there is no doubt that an understanding from a TESOL perspective adds significant breadth to this knowledge.

ASHA's Position Statement on providing ESL services in a school setting (1998, paragraph 1) notes the following: "It is the position of the American Speech-Language-Hearing Association (ASHA) that speech-language pathologists who possess the required knowledge and skills to provide English as a Second Language (ESL) instruction in school settings may provide direct ESL instruction. ESL instruction may require specialized academic preparation, and competencies in areas such as second language acquisition theory, comparative linguistics, and ESL methodologies, assessment, and practicum. Such specialized education may not be included in the education required for speech-language pathologists." While this statement is specifically designed to address working with children in a school setting, it stipulates that the qualifications necessary to do ESL work are not considered part of every SLP's training. By implication, SLPs who wish to help their non-native clients develop their overall English proficiency should ensure that they have the necessary knowledge base required to produce results and not merely superior skills in English as their L1. There are many more TESOL teachers than SLPs, and it is not difficult to find training programs and books of all types to develop professional skills. Many university extension departments and independent commercial programs offer live teacher-training courses, and there are a multitude online as well. In some cases, the

Because so many advanced non-native speakers have a very good grasp of English grammar, I found the grammar course requirements that were part of the TEFL certification program to be very helpful. I also invested in a series of grammar books by Betty Azar and found them to be quite useful, especially when researching answers to clients' complex grammar questions. The courses, workshops, and texts that focused on intonation and rhythm, stress, prosody, and word reductions have been key to helping clients achieve an American accent. Much of this information was initially new to me, but it became an integral part of therapy, often yielding dramatic results relatively quickly.

—Pat Chien

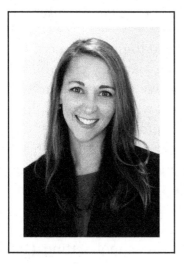

I have had to do a lot of self-study. This is an interdisciplinary service, so I have spent a lot of time looking into how other fields, such as ESL teachers, public speaking coaches, and voice and acting trainers, approach accent modification. I even decided to pursue a TESOL certificate so that I can better meet the needs of clients who have some specific grammar issues. I have also had to go back to some of my graduate and undergraduate books about phonetics and linguistics and take some additional courses in voice to help better understand how to manipulate resonance.

—Jamie Miller, M.S., CCC-SLP Advanced Accent Reduction

programs offer some type of TESOL certification, which should guarantee a strong foundation and may enhance clinicians' marketability. SLPs may also find that one or two courses in conjunction with some self-study will provide the necessary background. Appendix 11–1 lists materials for self-study, as well as resources for activities to use with clients.

## Additional Resources

An excellent starting point for both SLPs and students working in accent modification is the Facebook group SLPs in Accent Modification, which was started in 2014 by Autumn Bryant and is currently run by Paula Gallay. The group is only open to SLPs, SLPAs, and students who are working in accent modification. In Paula's words, the page was

Our purpose is to provide a community and resources for SLPs to connect, share, and enrich our practice of accent modification. A popular topic in our group is how start and grow an accent modification business, but members are also looking for practical information such as testing protocols, sample reports, and goals based on a client's first language.

—Paula Gallay

created "in response to the lack of online sites or chat rooms where SLPs could discuss accent modification without getting into the recurring argument of who was a better accent modification trainer—ESL teachers or SLPs. Actually, each can be a good trainer as each brings their knowledge and experience to the table." (Personal communication, 7/27/2018). There are several thousand members at this point, and it is an excellent meeting place for discussions and information. Professionals and students share ideas and resources and keep each other up-to-date on opportunities.

Another option to consider for anyone in private practice is the Corporate Speech Pathology Network (CORSPAN). According to its website (www.corspan.org) CORSPAN's mission is "to provide information, resources, networking, and client referrals to our members, while also promoting corporate speech pathology as a service to the public." The group was founded by Katie Schwartz in 1996 and it primarily focuses on SLPs who provide accent modification and public speaking training to corporations or individuals. There is an annual fee to join and membership is reserved for current and former holders of ASHA's Certificate of Clinical Competence. Members have access to a LISTSERV where they can discuss questions related to accent, private practice, and marketing, among

I would love to see accent modification become more widely sought after (and paid for!) by individuals and organizations. For that to happen, we, as accent modification training professionals, need to ensure that the general public and organizations recognize that the goal is not to diminish diversity, but rather celebrate diversity by allowing diverse minds and thoughts be successfully utilized, by using the right tools for clearer communication in the workplace. CORSPAN's mission is to provide networking, support, and resources to its members. Some ways in which CORSPAN executes its mission include regularly providing networking and mentoring opportunities, providing written marketing and educational resources for members to use in their own practice, providing free and low cost professional development and educational opportunities, and promoting corporate speech services to businesses and community organizations to increase awareness of corporate speech services availability and to build a global referral base for CORSPAN members.

—Sonia Sethi Kohli, MS, CCC-SLP, CORSPAN President

other topics. They also have access to resources and can create a membership profile that can be searched by potential clients seeking services.

For SLPs looking for an association dedicated to private practitioners that has a focus on the practical aspects of entrepreneurship, the American Academy of Private Practice in Speech Pathology and Audiology (AAPPSPA; http://www.aappspa.org) offers a range of services and benefits to its members. Membership in this non-profit organization, which was founded in 1964, is limited to SLPs or audiologists who already have an established private practice, but fledgling entrepreneurs are welcome as long as they are open for business and have started working with clients. In addition, both members and non-members alike are encouraged to attend their annual conference which is held every spring. AAPPSPA prides itself on providing support for the technical aspects of private practice, such as marketing, accounting, legal issues, and management, and they connect members through an online forum where practitioners exchange ideas on running their businesses and meeting the needs of their clients and communities.

The Institute of Language and Phonology (ILP) is often referred to as "Compton" after its founder Arthur J. Compton, who developed the PESL Program (Pronouncing English as a Second Language) in 1978. In 1985, he began to train SLPs in his methods, making this the longest running and perhaps most well-known accent modification training program for SLPs. The Institute is currently divided into three divisions: Research, Training, and Design and Technology. The ILP offers live workshops and training events, which provide ASHA-approved CEUs. Attendees who complete the coursework required to become certified trainers have access to testing and training materials, such as the P-ESL assessment discussed in Chapter 3. Many SLPs practicing in the field of accent modification have attended Compton trainings or use their methods and materials.

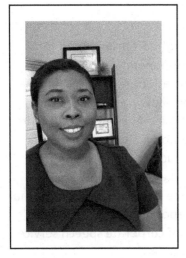

After I got my master's I started working for a school district. I worked with all grade levels, from Pre-K to 8th grade and discovered that I enjoyed working on speech sounds with the older kids more than working with the other goals or populations. However, I was growing weary of schools' undervaluation and mistreatment of SLP's and wanted to establish a way out. I took the Compton PESL course (twice) to introduce myself to working with adults on speech sounds, as this seemed the least intimidating bridge to leave schools. I already liked working with people I could carry on a conversation with and I already liked targeting phonemes and phonological patterns. After that I set up a website and began researching additional information on how to do accent modification and how to target prosody and other suprasegmentals.

—Autumn Bryant, MS, MA, CCC-SLP, Griffin Speech, Chartered

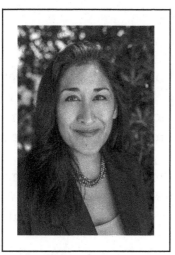

I've been interested in accent modification since I learned about it in graduate school. It seemed like a perfect marriage between my love for travel and other cultures and my passion for helping others communicate better. I took the Compton PESL Certification course and it expanded my initial spark of interest into a little burning flame that I carried with me through my years working as a school speech pathologist. When I made the decision to leave my school job, I knew I had to take the leap and try accent modification as a career.

—Indira Ryan, M.A., CCC-SLP San Diego Accent Specialists

Lorna Sikorski founded LDS & Associates (https://www.ldsassoc.com/) in 1987 to provide accent modification services to individuals and groups, and she currently specializes in providing training to SLPs looking to improve their skills in the field. In 2005, the LDS Online Trainer Center opened, where SLPs can receive training through distance learning. LDS & Associates also sells accent training materials, such as the MEEC (Mastering Effective English Communication) series, and their assessment the Proficiency in Oral English Communication (POEC) test discussed in Chapter 3.

There are many other programs that offer training for SLPs working in the field of accent modification. Some feature materials that can be purchased to use with clients, and many allow the name of their program to be used in marketing. Many of the programs also offer advice on how to establish a business, which make them excellent starting points for SLPs uncertain about the best way to begin. There are also many resources available for entrepreneurs in general. According to its website, https://www.score.org/, SCORE is "America's premier source of free and confidential small business advice for entrepreneurs and small businesses, is a nonprofit resource partner with the US. Small Business Administration (SBA)." (Paragraph 1). It is a 501(c)(3) organization (nonprofit) that offers mentoring, workshops, online business tools, and other resources for entrepreneurs. The U.S. Small Business Administration (SBA) https://www.sba.gov/ also features a number of useful resources designed for planning and launching a business.

The best resource I have found is other people—linking up with someone who is practicing accent modification and observing what they do.

—Julie Cunningham

# University Clinics

## Student Clinicians

Accent modification is often provided by graduate student clinicians under the supervision of licensed SLPs at university clinics. In some clinics, a supervisor (generally one who works primarily with adults) oversees students working with accent clients who come in on a case-by-case basis, while other clinics have a full program which is regularly open to clients. In both scenarios, clients are often students or faculty from the university, but clinics may also be open to the public. A survey of graduate clinics offering accent modification conducted by Schmidt & Sullivan (2003) found that 97% served students, with 28% serving them exclusively. Some students also receive supervised accent modification training off campus, although this is less common.

Graduate students are often excited to have the chance to work with non-native clients, but they may be apprehensive since they often feel they do not have the training for this type of work. It is important for students to realize that they are not alone; some veteran SLPs entering the field of accent modification have the same apprehensions. Students must rely on the hard work, talent, instincts, and personal strengths that got them into graduate school, and then devote themselves to bridging the gap between the strong foundation they have in phonetics and language acquisition and the additional knowledge they need to work with non-disordered adults acquiring the phonology of a second language. I have supervised many graduate students in accent modification and have always been impressed by their diligence and dedication. Students are creative and highly motivated, and within a short timeframe, they are able to produce excellent results. These students exit the program with knowledge and experience that can shape their futures since the basic techniques involved in accent modification, such as modeling, feedback, and generalization training apply to all of the work SLPs do. In addition, the insight gained from working with accent modification clients will be immensely beneficial when working with non-native speakers in any setting.

---

If a graduate program offers an accent modification clinic, I think students should take advantage of it. It's another side of speech therapy that students can learn about and eventually pursue as professionals. Not only can they use what they learn in accent modification to help clients improve their accents, but they can apply what they've learned to other clinical settings as well. When I found out I would be working with accent clients, I felt pretty nervous because my first semester working with them was also my first semester of clinic. Over time, I learned so much about my clients and the different methods I could use to help them improve their accents that by the end of the semester, I not only felt more confident and comfortable in clinic, but I was sad to see my clients go.

—Jessica Williams

# The Accent and Communication Training Program at SDSU

San Diego State University's Accent and Communication Training (ACT) Program, which was founded in the fall of 1992, is an example of a graduate training program in accent modification. The following is a description of our program with the hope that it can provide a useful model for others. The program currently operates twice a year, during the fall and spring semesters. Each semester, four graduate student clinicians are assigned by the clinic director to work under a licensed faculty supervisor. Figure 11–1 shows four graduate clinicians in front of the SDSU clinic at the beginning of the semester. Before the client sessions begin, students undergo approximately 10 to 12 hours of preparatory training. In these sessions, the supervisor and student clinicians discuss the principles of accent modification and review useful techniques. Potential clients are reviewed and eight are selected for training. Some of the time spent during these first few weeks relates to program management since schedules have to be created and client preferences need to be factored into planning.

One important feature of the program is that clients are normally offered only one complete semester to attend. In private practice, training generally continues until the client decides to discontinue services, or if there is a mutual agreement that a plateau has been reached. The goal in developing the ACT program was to provide a good overview of English phonology and to focus on the key areas that would provide the most rapid improvement in communicative effectiveness for each client. We allow only one semester per client because if clients repeated the program, it would be difficult to provide the general information in a fresh way, and there would be a risk that continuing work on the same targets for several semesters in a row might make clients feel they were in a rut. When working with native-speaking children on articulation there is an expectation of

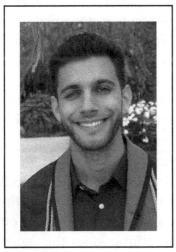

I was very excited when I found out I would be working with accent clients. It was a great experience and I would do it all over again. It's important to be flexible and understanding, and the biggest challenge for me was finding new materials and being creative. I think I figured out my way as the semester progressed though. At the end of the semester, I felt like I made a difference with my clients. I connected with them and provided technical feedback to help them improve their accent. Build a strong connection and then the rest will fall into place!

—Jordan Mantel, Graduate Clinician

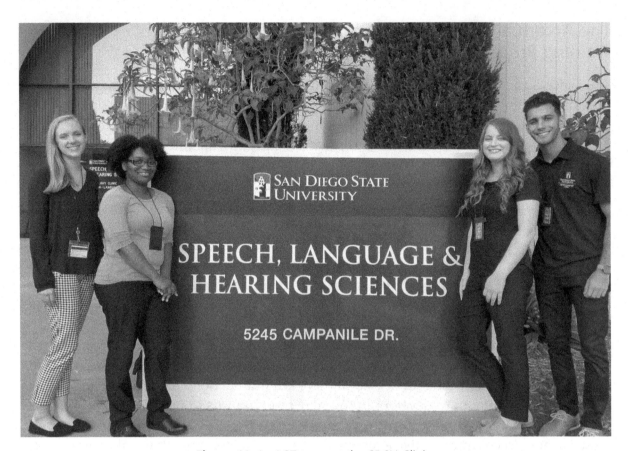

**Figure 11–1.** ACT team at the SDSU Clinic.

remediation, and therefore, it makes sense to continue working on targets until they are acquired, but with non-native speakers there is generally no expectation of a specific final outcome. This one shot approach also focuses clients since they know that the number of sessions is limited, and it allows the program to serve more clients.

In the past, there was a nominal fee charged to the clients based on whether they were students, faculty, or community members, but currently services are provided on a donation basis. Clients are often generous with their support because they realize the incredible value of this type of service. Most clients come to the program by word of mouth or through some light recruitment efforts undertaken by the supervisor or students. In some cases, an email is sent out to department chairs to attract faculty or graduate assistants as clients. In selecting clients, the preference is for clients who have advanced communication skills in all aspects of English with the exception of phonology, but clients generally arrive with a wide range of abilities. Diversity of languages is also prized since this tends to make group sessions more dynamic. All clients are adults who come to the program voluntarily, and they tend to be highly motivated to make changes to their pronunciation. Clients who are interested in attending the program fill out a simple one-page application which asks for basic contact information, the languages they speak, where they are from, and their age of arrival in the United States. They are also asked to

**Table 11–1.** ACT Program Format

| Week | Day 1 | Day 2 |
|------|-------|-------|
| 1 | Hour 1 (Individual)<br>Clinician A with Client 1<br>Clinician B with Client 2<br>Clinician C with Client 3<br>Clinician D with Client 4 | Hour 1 (Individual)<br>Clinician A with Client 1<br>Clinician B with Client 2<br>Clinician C with Client 3<br>Clinician D with Client 4 |
| | Hour 2 (Individual)<br>Clinician A with Client 5<br>Clinician B with Client 6<br>Clinician C with Client 7<br>Clinician D with Client 8 | Hour 2 (Individual)<br>Clinician A with Client 5<br>Clinician B with Client 6<br>Clinician C with Client 7<br>Clinician D with Client 8 |
| 2 | Hour 1 (Individual)<br>Clinician A with Client 1<br>Clinician B with Client 2<br>Clinician C with Client 3<br>Clinician D with Client 4 | Hour 1 (Pairs)<br>Clinician A with Clients 1 & 5<br>Clinician B with Clients 2 & 6<br>Clinician C with Clients 3 & 7<br>Clinician D with Clients 4 & 8 |
| | Hour 2 (Individual)<br>Clinician A with Client 5<br>Clinician B with Client 6<br>Clinician C with Client 7<br>Clinician D with Client 8 | Hour 2 (Group)<br>Clinicians A–D with Clients 1–8 |

rate their English listening, speaking, grammar, and pronunciation abilities. In keeping with the desire to develop an awareness that accents are normal, there are no detailed questions about personal or medical history, but there is one question that asks the applicants if they have any communication difficulties in their native language.

The current version of the program has evolved over the last few years based on clinician ideas and client feedback. The program runs for about 11 weeks each semester and clients come for a two-hour slot twice weekly. On most days, clients come for individual sessions for either the first or second hour, but for one day every two weeks they are paired up for a one-hour session, and then they have a group session for the second hour. Twice-weekly training sessions appear to be typical throughout the country; Schmidt and Sullivan (2003) found in their survey that 65% of the graduate programs providing accent modification had biweekly sessions with only 3% seeing the clients more often (in intensive programs that were short-term). Table 11–1 illustrates what a two-week section of the semester looks like.

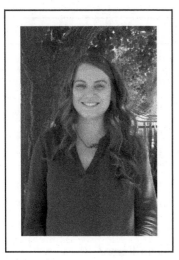

I really enjoyed group sessions where all the clients were able to interact with each other and discuss common challenges they have faced with English pronunciation. Seeing them work so hard every session inspired me to work harder as a clinician and a student. I really looked forward to my sessions every week and seeing their improvement at the end of the semester was the most rewarding part.

—Natalie Spieckerman, Graduate Clinician

Group sessions are extremely valuable for several reasons. First, they create a sense of community for the clients, so that they can share their experiences of having an accent and the progress they are making during the training. Second, it allows for dynamic activities that benefit from group work. Often this involves work on suprasegmentals through role plays, pair work, or games. Last, having clients in group allows all of the clinicians to get to know each client, and that builds a more cohesive program. For example, when a clinician discusses a client during a team meeting, other team members have a much better understanding since they have worked with the client as well.

The first session of the program is conducted with the group as a whole and consists of a general introduction aimed at developing clients' awareness of the key issues involved in accent. Clinicians generally discuss the critical period, the importance of effective communication as opposed to a native-like accent, and some of the key terminology. One of the key functions of the first session is to give clinicians a chance to listen to the clients speech since they are always new each semester. After the session, clinicians and their supervisor work together to determine which clients should be paired together and which clinician will work with each pair. The primary criterion for this determination is the overall English level of each client because large differences in ability could lead to frustration during the paired sessions. Generally, it is easiest to find the clients with the lowest level of English ability and pair them together first; matching on overall ability is less important for relatively high-level L2 speakers. Native language, age, gender, personality and other factors also play a role in matching pairs. Once the pairs are established, clinicians work together to determine who will take which pair. One other important factor is time preference. Clients are told that they should be available from 4 to 6 p.m., but they can choose a time preference for either 4:00 or 5:00 p.m. for their individual sessions.

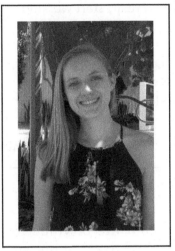

Don't be afraid to keep reassessing your goals and your clients' needs throughout the semester; if you notice something in their speech, don't be afraid to immediately pursue it and probe it. Do a thorough assessment, and make sure that you identify in what contexts they have linguistic and/or phonological differences. Involve them in their training, and make sure that you prioritize what they would like you to prioritize. However, also use your expertise to identify what it is that stands out to you and may benefit most from training.

—Hannah Grant, Graduate Clinician

After the first group session, clients return for their first individual meeting and an assessment is conducted. The assessment generally takes most or all of the first session, and clinicians are discouraged from extending the assessment into the second meeting. The general procedures used are outlined in Chapter 3 on assessment. Clinicians develop goals and goal areas for the clients based on their assessments, but they are also encouraged to adapt throughout the program to provide the maximum benefit during the semester.

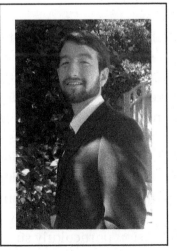

The most rewarding part of working with accent clients was twofold. First, seeing my clients successfully produce a sound for the first time and how happy they were to know that they were succeeding was very rewarding. Second, seeing the confidence boost clients received from the sessions and seeing how satisfied they were with their own progress made me feel as if I had truly helped out another person. The clients are highly motivated, value your experience and input, and are very grateful for the training you provide.

—Benjamin Zarotsky, Graduate Clinician

Have fun and learn as much as you can. This is a good opportunity to really start working with clients from a wide variety of backgrounds if you haven't yet. Also, listen to your clients and get to know them. Find out their strengths and weaknesses and use that to find the best way to improve the clarity and naturalness of their speech. Finally, keep your sessions client-centered, work on targets that are relevant to their everyday lives, and try to provide them with opportunities to practice what they've been learning in broader contexts (e.g., using role play scenarios).

—Jessica Williams

Once the program begins, group sessions address areas that are of value to all clients. This can include segmental targets that are problematic for most of the group, but commonly the focus is on suprasegmentals, since they are most likely to benefit all clients. Individual sessions are designed to provide extended practice in specific areas that clients need to work on to become more effective communicators.

Clinicians create lesson plans before each session and write notes afterwards. The supervisor monitors each session and provides written and oral feedback to help develop the students' skills. There are weekly staff meetings to provide general feedback and address any concerns. Midterm and final conferences with the graduate students are designed to review their strengths and help them improve any areas that need development.

During the final session, students give their clients a final report that outlines the work they did during the semester and provides some issues clients can focus on in the future. These reports will most likely be read by the clients alone; therefore, every effort is made to reduce jargon, explain any technical terms, and use examples. In the final group session, clients share their experiences and future goals, which creates a powerful sense of closure. After this, there is a chance to chat informally to wrap up.

## Group Work

There are many advantages to running group sessions, whether they are in a university clinic setting or in a private accent program, and this section provides some tips for creating effective opportunities for clients to benefit. The key advantage involves the change in dynamics that come about when non-native speakers work together. Clients begin to feel a sense of community with others who face similar challenges, and this is an essential way for them to share their knowledge and help each other progress. In the traditional education model, teachers were the source of knowledge and students were the receptacles, but the modern focus is on collaborative learning, where students and teachers share in the discovery of ideas. Speech pathology also has a tradition of promoting a model in which clinicians are authority figures, and when dealing with clients who have disabilities it is hard to avoid making this impression particularly strong.

In the world of accent modification, clinicians typically have a native accent and a great deal of knowledge, but in this case, clients are not disordered and they have much knowledge to share. The group experience is especially effective at nudging this balance a little more in the clients' direction.

Clinicians are advised, therefore, to limit the amount of explaining and lecturing during group sessions and make an effort to create multiple interactions. If we think in terms of practice opportunities, group sessions have a clear advantage over individual sessions. Clinicians should always be mindful of maintaining a good clinician to client talking ratio, and the easiest way to accomplish this is to have clients work together in pairs or small groups. When clients interact with each other and the clinician monitors the interaction, clients have many opportunities to take ownership of their pronunciation work. Clinicians often feel that they must be involved in every exchange, but in reality, there is much value in allowing clients to practice and coach each other while the clinician listens and steps in when concerns arise. SLPs also like to see results, but often in the world of accent modification we plant seeds by increasing awareness, and the actual change in speech patterns may occur at a later date. We need to allow some time for clients to work through ideas and process the information presented to them. Clinicians can introduce an activity, then pair off students, monitor, take notes, and at the end, provide some feedback to the group as a whole.

A powerful technique in both group and individual sessions is elicitation. Clinicians and teachers often feel that they need to provide all of the information and answers to students, but in reality, there is power in allowing students to discover their own answers. If we take the example of the rules for the regular past tense endings, clients may retain the information better if given the three types of endings and asked to determine the rules. Clinicians can provide some direction and use scaffolding to guide clients to the answer, but if clients are involved in the process they will be more engaged than if they are simply provided with the rules.

# In Their Own Words

To conclude this chapter, clinicians who have entered the field of accent modification describe how they got started and where it has led them, as well as some of the many rewards and challenges they have discovered along the way.

## Career Paths

It is extremely rare for SLPs to complete their clinical fellowship year in a setting where they provide full-time accent modification services. In almost every case, SLPs who are currently working with non-native speakers started their careers in more traditional settings and then decided to branch out to work with non-native speakers.

I'm a practicing speech-language pathologist working with the adult population in the hospital, acute rehab, and outpatient settings. I taught English in the Czech Republic in my mid-20s, and I really enjoyed working with clients who were from a different culture. After returning to the U.S., I knew I wanted to continue working with those same types of people, but I didn't know how. Then I discovered accent modification, and it just clicked.

—Julie Cunningham

While working at a private practice I suddenly realized that I was no longer feeling fulfilled working with a pool of clients that skewed heavily toward children aged 2–18. When I happened to be assigned adult clients with voice and fluency issues, I realized that I really preferred working with adults at this stage of my life. Things crystallized even more when I was asked to pull together materials in order to work with several non-native speakers who had requested accent modification. Even though I lacked the materials and the confidence to modify their accents, the work was energizing and the clients were content with a "let's figure this out together" approach. All of this led to a major career change starting with an application to UCSD's TEFL program, which I attended part-time while continuing to work in private practice. I attended multiple accent modification workshops and anything else that was available at the time. I decided to build my own private practice which grew slowly but steadily over the years.

—Pat Chien

After graduate school, I became a school-based SLP and worked with elementary and high school students. I really enjoyed working with them but I wanted to have more control in my career and try something new. I learned so much that helped prepare me for my accent modification work and I feel very grateful for my years as a school SLP. I also did volunteer work in accent modification when I lived in Tasmania. Their vocational school, TAFE, has an adult English program for immigrants and refugees and I was able to do pronunciation work with them. It was a fun challenge to learn and then teach my students an Australian English accent!

—Indira Ryan

I have always been interested in different languages and cultures, and in addition to speaking multiple languages, I have always had an interest in learning different accents and speaking mannerisms. Also, throughout my life, I have had the fortunate opportunity to interact with and assist with linguistic and cultural adjustment for many immigrants and visitors from foreign countries that come to the USA, which also played an important part in leading me down this path.

—Sonia Sethi Kohli

## Challenges

Leaving the well-known traditional pathways takes courage, and many SLPs report that they feel they have to discover a great deal on their own. In addition, developing a successful private practice involves expertise in areas such as marketing and bookkeeping that may not come naturally to many SLPs.

---

One of the biggest challenges is finding workable schedules for each individual. Many clients work long hours, so there are often appointments made, then broken and rescheduled. Non-compliance can be an issue, especially with homework assignments. When clients have busy work schedules plus families, finding the time to practice can be a huge challenge. Many of my clients use our recordings to practice in the car on the way to and from work. Financial issues can also be a problem but, with experience, I have worked out different payment plans and eventually have become more comfortable with the financial aspects of running a business.

—Pat Chien

---

Scheduling clients is the biggest problem. I usually have to see accent improvement clients late in the afternoon or on Saturday mornings. Another challenge is that clients may have comprehension problems that become apparent after a few sessions, and sometimes an accent is not the problem.

—Steve Glance

---

For me the biggest challenges are 1) knowing how to price this service, 2) finding enough clients who want this service, and 3) getting busy working professionals to do their homework.

—Autumn Bryant

---

I think learning the business side of things has been very challenging. There is just so much to know about marketing, bookkeeping, websites, and the list goes on. It's challenging for me to manage my time well, balancing all of the many hats I have to wear as a small business owner, as well as family and personal time.

—Jamie Miller

One of my biggest challenges has been learning how to become a businesswoman. There are so many components that have nothing to do with accent modification involved in turning a passion into a successful career—marketing, bookkeeping, technology, etcetera—and unless you have strong business acumen, it can feel overwhelming. Another challenge has been finding adequate training in accent modification. I've found that many training programs are either too limited in scope or can be prohibitively expensive.

—Indira Ryan

## Rewards

When asked about the rewards of working in the field of accent modification, the answer is almost universal—it is the clients. SLPs are exceptionally caring, and helping these clients achieve their communication goals is the most oft-cited benefit.

I really find it rewarding to see my clients achieve success and truly reach their professional potential. Many times, the wealth of information and ideas that these professionals possess are never really fully recognized or are "lost in translation," simply due to (nonmedical- or developmental) communication challenges related to pronunciation, cross-cultural communication differences, or both. I thoroughly enjoy the experience of setting goals with my client, witnessing them achieve those professional goals, and also witnessing my clients actually realize that they have achieved their goals, giving them the confidence to challenge themselves even more to achieve their highest potential.

—Sonia Sethi Kohli

Because I've always been interested in cross-cultural experiences and have been fortunate enough to travel extensively around the world, the one-on-one meetings and relationship building that's part and parcel of accent reduction therapy is a huge plus for me. The problem solving aspects of the work also appeal to me; the "cracking the code" of a particular accent, followed by formulation of a game plan to make the most progress in the most efficient manner. The work is never humdrum, as two individuals from the same town in the same province of the same country might have different issues. There's definitely a strong intellectual component to the work, as the practitioner pulls information from every corner of his or her experience in order to serve the client. There are often multiple layers of accent that must be teased out during the initial diagnostic phase. Because most clients are highly motivated adult learners, there is none of the cajoling and bribery that go along with working with a juvenile population. Although there are often enormous individual differences in the rates of progress, most of the time there is steady progress, which is rewarding to both practitioner and client.

—Pat Chien

I feel like the accent modification clients are truly my people. They are me if I knew a second language as proficiently as they do. They're smart, savvy, motivated, and ambitious. I love helping them boost their confidence and moving them closer to their career goals, as many of them choose this service to help themselves advance in their fields.

—Autumn Bryant

I remember how I felt when I misspoke or didn't understand something when I lived abroad: disconnected and isolated. So I find it extremely rewarding to help my clients feel more at home in the United States when they feel more comfortable and experience less frustration speaking in English. One of my clients told me that she used to feel shy when she was talking to Americans and that she became more confident and social after having accent modification sessions. Another client regularly used an American nickname because he was tired of repeating his name to people. When I taught him a modified way to say his name that was more intelligible to Americans, he was so happy to give up his nickname.

—Indira Ryan

Speech-language pathology, no matter what setting or population you're working with, is about helping people become successful communicators. It's what I love about our field. In that way, accent modification is no different. But what I love about accent modification is being a part of the success story for people who are on their way up in this country. We get to be working in the background to help create unity and to build bridges of successful communication. By removing the obstacle of intelligibility, we are empowering people to be seen for who they really are and doing our little part in the world to help people see that we really aren't that different. I love to see how clear and confident communication opens doors to career and social opportunities for people who could otherwise be isolated or marginalized.

—Jamie Miller

# References

American Speech-Language-Hearing Association (ASHA) Multicultural Issues Board. (1998). *Provision of instruction in English as a second language by speech-language pathologists in school settings* (Position statement). Retrieved from https://www.asha.org/policy/PS1998-00102/

Schmidt, A. M., & Sullivan, S. (2003). Clinical training in foreign accent modification: A national survey. *Contemporary Issues in Communication Science and Disorders, 30,* 127–135.

# 11–1

# Accent Modification Resource Sheet

## Overviews

Celce-Murcia, M., Brinton, D., & Goodwin, J. M. (2010). *Teaching pronunciation: A course book and reference guide* (2nd ed.). New York, NY: Cambridge University Press.

Derwing, T., & Munro, M. (2015). *Pronunciation fundamentals: Evidence-based perspectives for L2 teaching and research*. Philadelphia, PA: John Benjamins Publishing Company.

Ehrlich, S., & Peter, A. (2013). *Teaching American English pronunciation*. Oxford, UK: Oxford University Press.

Kimble-Fry, A., & ClearSpeak (2001). *Perfect pronunciation: A guide for trainers and self-help students*. Sydney, AU: ClearSpeak Pty Ltd.

Kreidler, C. W. (1989). *The pronunciation of English: A course book in phonology*. Oxford, UK: Blackwell.

Murphy, J., & University of Michigan Press (2017). *Teaching the pronunciation of English: Focus on whole courses*. Ann Arbor, MI: University of Michigan Press.

Murphy, J. (2017). *The Routledge handbook of contemporary English pronunciation*. London, UK: Routledge.

Reed, M., & Levis, J. (2015). *The handbook of English pronunciation*. Malden, MA: Wiley-Blackwell.

## Coursebooks for Clients

Cook, A. (2012). *American accent training* (3rd ed.). Hauppauge, NY: Barron's.

Grant, L. (2016). *Well said: Pronunciation for clear communication* (4th ed.). Boston, MA: Heinle & Heinle Publishers.

Lujan, B. (2016). *The American accent guide* (3rd ed.). Salt Lake City, UT: Lingual Arts.

Meyers, C. M., & Holt, S. (2001). *Pronunciation for success: Student workbook*. Burnsville, MN: Aspen Productions.

Miller, S. (2006). *Targeting pronunciation: Communicating clearly in English* (2nd ed.). Boston, MA: Thomson Heinle.

Mosjin, L. (2016). *Mastering the American accent* (2nd ed.). Hauppauge, NY: Barron's.

# Social Media

SLPs in Accent Modification Facebook page https://www.facebook.com/groups/543299812453471/
CORSPAN https://www.facebook.com/findaspeechtrainer/
The Accent Authority https://www.facebook.com/The-Accent-Authority-232361463589909/

# Internet Resources

CORSPAN http://www.corspan.org/
Rachel's English https://www.youtube.com/user/rachelsenglish
Jennifer-English Pronunciation https://www.youtube.com/watch?v=qMM_hwyHxaI&list=PL0B58
    DCD9199D5668
English Accent Coach https://www.englishaccentcoach.com/index.aspx
Speech Accent Archive http://accent.gmu.edu/
Pronunciation for Teachers http://www.pronunciationforteachers.com/
Teaching Pronunciation: A handbook for teachers and trainers
https://helenfraser.com.au/wp-content/uploads/HF-Handbook.pdf
American Academy of Private Practice in Speech Pathology and Audiology https://www.aappspa.org
Voice and Speech Trainers Association https://www.vasta.org/

# Journal

*Journal of Second Language Pronunciation.* John Benjamins. https://benjamins.com/#catalog/journals
    /jslp/main

# Index

Note: Page numbers in **bold** reference non-text material.